PRAISE FOR
THE ONE-MINUTE CURE

"One of the best books on health I read in 40 years"

"Wow, this was one of the best books on health I read in my 40 years of existence. It was very thorough, well laid out and something that I will share with all my friends and associates. I started using your recommended dosage right away and you are right, I feel great and I know and feel that my body will be disease-free. Thanks again for being part of the solution to making our world a better and safer place for all man and woman kind." — Jacques A., Atlanta, Georgia

"Every household must have this book"

"I was very skeptical and actually thought this one-minute cure was nothing but a scam when I watched the Cancer Cure video on YouTube. I bought the book anyway because I wanted to expose the book's author as just another con artist preying on people's fear of disease. But when I read the book, it radically changed my belief as to how cancer, heart disease, AIDS and other diseases come about, and are cured. Cavanaugh offers credible arguments, backed by solid evidence, that this one-minute cure is indeed the world's answer to cancer. Every household must have this book." -- Orson Dillard, Boston, Massachusetts

"This book is worth far more than its weight in gold!"

"I watched family members (mom and brother) die of cancer in recent years. No matter how well-meaning the doctors were, they couldn't help because all they were taught in med school was to prescribe surgery, chemotherapy or radiation, none of which cured my mom and brother but maybe hastened their deaths. The One-Minute Cure has really opened my eyes to the hidden agenda of Big Pharma that wants to keep us sick because they earn more profits from our ongoing diseases.

"But the promise of a one-minute cure ... although I wanted to believe it with all my heart, seemed too good to be true. I nearly passed up reading this book, but I didn't want to wait till my husband, children or loved ones die of cancer, only to realize too late that the one-minute cure could've saved their lives. So I read the book from cover to cover and discovered that it's worth far more than its weight in gold! My family will be using the one-minute cure for the rest of our lives." -- Lucille Wilkinson, Ann Arbor, Michigan

"Wow! is the only way to describe this book"

"When I started reading the book ... I discovered the profound impact that the information in the book would have in my life, as well as the lives of countless others. All I could say was "Wow!" The greatest value I received from this book is that the author successfully compiled all the relevant research regarding the therapeutic use of the natural oxygenating substance and put it into one slim volume that can be understood, appreciated and used by the general population. As someone who considers himself knowledgeable about natural health therapies, products and services, I highly recommend this outstanding book." -- Bruce Lloyd, New York, NY

"The definitive answer to disease"

"I've never been this impressed with any health breakthrough that has surfaced in the natural health arena in the last few decades. The One-Minute Cure, which is validated by volumes of irrefutable scientific evidence, may quite possibly be the panacea that we've all been looking for. I believe it's the definitive answer to the cause, prevention and cure of a great many diseases that plague the world today." -- M. Chancellor, Los Angeles, California

"I experienced an EPIPHANY after reading this wonderful, wonderful book!"

"When I came across the website of The One-Minute Cure, I suspected that this 'secret to healing virtually all diseases' was probably oxygen or an alkaline pH ... and curiosity made me order the book. I am SO THANKFUL I did! After I finished reading this book ... I had an epiphany! I realized that with this book, I already HAVE the cure for everything! I've been spreading the word to everyone and telling them that The One-Minute Cure is a necessary addition to their health library. It's a wonderful, wonderful book that will help people wake up in many ways." -- Libby Lervik, Port Hardy, British Columbia

"This book is a gift to mankind!"

"I almost clicked away from The One-Minute Cure website, almost jumping to the conclusion that it was just another commercial enterprise wanting to make a fast buck from desperate people. But I was too curious to know what the heck this 'natural oxygenating substance' was that they were talking about. So I ordered the book, and I'm so very glad I did. Sincere thanks to the author for bringing this important information to so many of us who are in such great need of it. It's truly a gift to mankind!" -- Tamara W., Miami, Florida

"...the spearhead of a health revolution!"

"Madison, I read your book straight through and have already emailed friends about it. Your work comes at a good time ... We are living in a very wicked world. I see your book as the spearhead of a health revolution, which I have been preaching to deaf ears for 15 years or more." -- John I., Marsascala, Malta

"This book has had a PROFOUND impact on me"

"As soon as I got the book, I began to read it and haven't been able to stop until I have finished it! The first thing that has come to my mind is "EVERYONE OUGHT TO READ THIS BOOK!" Your book has really had a profound impact on me." -- D. Garcia, Guardiola de Font Rubi, Spain

"Compelling evidence of a veritable cure-all..."

"One-Minute Cure contains thoroughly researched material that indeed offers compelling evidence of a veritable cure-all for all diseases. Unlike other self-proclaimed 'cures' promoted by others in the name of profiteering, the author clearly has no other agenda than to bring this hope of healing to every man, woman and child who's in need of it." -- Cheryl Jeter, Alternative Frontier Newsletter

"The magical miracle cure for virtually all disease!"

"I bought 3 copies of this book ... and have been applying the advice as described in the book. Now 8 years later, I have not had one cold, flu, viral infection, indigestion, or any other one of those ailments. My energy levels are high, eyesight 20/20 and basically body functions as if I was a 40 year old (am 70+). Reading this book and applying the recommendations is THE cure for people's health in this century. I give this book a 5-Star rating, because I myself feel as the shining example, of how healthy one can feel, after following the wisdom, made public in this book." -- M. Ron, Amazon Verified Purchaser of The-One-Minute-Cure book.

The One-Minute Cure

The Secret to Healing
Virtually All Diseases

SECOND EDITION

By Madison Cavanaugh

The One-Minute Cure: The Secret to Healing Virtually All Diseases
SECOND EDITION

Publisher:

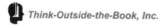 *Think-Outside-the-Book, Inc.*

8465 W. Sahara Avenue, Suite 111-497
Summerlin, Nevada
USA 89117
http://www.ThinkOutsideTheBook.com

Printed in the U.S.A.

Table of Contents

AUTHOR'S INTRODUCTION TO THE SECOND EDITION

When *The One-Minute Cure* book was first published in 2008 — a year before it became a No. 1 bestselling health book for several years — I never imagined how rapidly it would grow in popularity worldwide. Over the past decade, the one-minute therapy presented in this book has gone from being an obscure curiosity in the alternative health community to a globally recognized health option for healing virtually all diseases.

A growing number of medical and healthcare practitioners have begun to appreciate the merits of this drugless therapy, and some have even acknowledged it as "the greatest healing miracle of all time." Indeed, as the dangers of standard medical treatments have become painfully apparent and the costs of medical care treatments have skyrocketed beyond reach, the modern day world has yearned for a viable, reliable and sustainable natural "medicine" suitable for most ailments—one which is accessible and affordable to all. I'm overjoyed to acknowledge that the one-minute therapy discussed in this book has stepped in to meet that need.

In the past 13 years, I have received thousands of letters, reports, testimonials and e-mails from readers describing how the *The One-Minute Cure* has helped them overcome a wide variety of health conditions, ailments and diseases ranging from asthma to diabetes to heart disease. Perhaps this is why this therapy has been dubbed by many as the panacea of our time.

More specifically, people from all over the world have reported that they've been able to heal themselves or their loved ones of **cancer**, and as such, the one-minute cure has become the preferred natural therapy for many who are battling cancer. Perhaps the most stunning demonstration of how this simple therapy helps overcome cancer is this: If one were to place a cancerous tumor the size of a golf ball into a bowl containing the natural oxygenating substance which is the centerpiece of this therapy, the tumor would start shrinking within minutes—and will completely disappear in a matter of hours!

This phenomenon occurs because most microbes, viruses, harmful bacteria, disease microorganisms and pathogens are anaerobic—which means they thrive only in environments where oxygen is absent. Conversely, when they're placed in an environment where oxygen is abundant, they cannot survive. It stands to reason that once the natural oxygenating substance prescribed in this book is introduced into the human body, the body becomes *uninhabitable by cancer.*

Countless testimonials of people getting healed of cancer—even late-stage or terminal cancer—within weeks, have given most people the impression that the one-minute cure is a therapy focused solely on healing cancer. Of course, that health benefit alone would make this therapy priceless—especially since it costs only 1½ cents per day to self-administer. However, the one-minute cure is much more than a therapeutic option for cancer. The natural oxygenating substance described in this book has such far-reaching and broad spectrum effectiveness in healing an extensive number of diseases—from the common cold to acute or chronic health conditions, autoimmune and degenerative diseases, inflammatory diseases and virtually any ailment, whether mild, severe or life-threatening. Sprinkled throughout the pages of this 2nd edition are the extraordinary stories of real people who have conquered every manner of disease using the one-minute cure.

When the subject of updating and revising *The One-Minute Cure* book was proposed, one had to wonder, "Is there anything new to add or write that would fit into the scope of a second edition?" My unequivocal answer is "Yes!" In fact, this 2nd edition is long overdue. The delay in its publication will become apparent as you read the rest of this chapter.

Although the basic one-minute therapy presented in the first edition remains unchanged and has withstood the test of time, there is now an abundance of new information and compelling scientific research (more than 91,000 studies) supporting the original premise. There are also numerous anecdotal case studies validating the success of the one-minute therapy on a wide variety of health conditions.

Upon writing this 2nd edition, I reviewed the books and research studies cited in the first edition, retained references to those studies that are still valid and evergreen, and have also added a wealth of research and scientific references, including an expanded Bibliography for those who wish to further their education on the subject matter. I have also included a Resources section and answers to the most Frequently Asked Questions I've received from readers over the years.

Furthermore, I've added a few new sections to this book, the most important of which may be the introduction of a way to overcome the greatest health crisis mankind has faced in a hundred years.

With the arrival of the COVID-19 pandemic, the remarkable power of the one-minute therapy becomes even more significant—not just life-changing but also world-changing! COVID-19 and all its variants have become a chilling presence in the world's health landscape—and will probably affect the way we live on our planet for decades to come. Chapter 5 presents a little-known method for administering the natural oxygenating substance that one doctor referred to as *"the single most effective intervention for those who have acute COVID-19."* Another doctor has successfully treated over 207 COVID-19 patients with this same mode of administration and even published a case paper about this treatment.

The reason for the delay in the publication of this 2nd edition now becomes apparent. I believe that this edition has come to be published for such a time as this—a time when the world is filled with uncharted and unprecedented dangers to human health and life, COVID-19 being only one of them.

When I wrote the first edition of this book back in 2008, my goal was to "plant" this book—as one would plant seeds—into every household in the world. That's because there isn't a man, woman or child who cannot benefit from the health secret contained herein—a secret that is not only simple but also profound in its far-reaching implications. This expanded edition underscores the importance of the fundamental chemistry of oxygen, water and hydrogen peroxide—and when you awaken to that truth you'll realize that **you will never be sick again.**

~ CHAPTER ONE ~

The information you are about to read in this book will not only *shock* you, but also *anger* and *excite* you at the same time. It will shock you because the simple therapy presented herein may be the closest thing to a *panacea* that you've ever encountered, and yet it has been deliberately suppressed by those who care less about protecting people's health than they do about their own financial interests. It will make you angry because you might have relatives, friends and loved ones who have suffered unnecessarily from preventable diseases, or even died, because this information has not been disseminated as vigilantly as it should have been. And lastly, it will excite you because the simple therapy which is the subject of this book may well be what its supporters call "the world's greatest healing miracle of all time."

If you are like most people, you probably find it hard to believe that any **single** therapy, substance or element could have such a far-reaching and broad spectrum efficacy when it comes to curing diseases. You have every reason to be skeptical. You might be thinking, 'How could anything so simple actually be the answer to all our complex health problems?'

The fact is, simple concepts are often the most powerful ones—and yet usually the most ignored. This is particularly true in the healthcare field. Over the last seven centuries, we as a society have been programmed to regard the curing or healing of disease as a perplexing and complicated science that is best left in the hands of medical practitioners. As a result, we've come to rely almost exclusively on the information that is dispensed to us by doctors and health care providers who are themselves usually uninformed about alternative healing options that may be more efficacious for treating diseases than the standard medical treatments consisting of drugs, surgery, radiation or other therapies.

What you're about to learn from this book is a simple, inexpensive therapy that can be self-administered at home in less than a minute—and costs about 1½ cents per day. An estimated 15,000 European medical doctors, naturopaths and homeopaths have provided this powerful therapy to over 10 million people over the past 80 years to treat over 50 different diseases. In the U.S., a comparatively smaller number of doctors and health practitioners provide this therapy. According to the American College for Advancement in Medicine (ACAM) and International Oxidative Medicine Association (IOMA), less than 500 U.S. health practitioners have this therapy available, although these lists are far from exhaustive. There are more than 91,000 studies that scientifically validate the efficacy of this therapy (more than double the 40,000 studies in existence at the time of this book's first edition). Yet, this therapy is still relatively unknown in the U.S. because of reasons that will become clear as you read the rest of this book.

Before I reveal what that therapy is, it is necessary to present an abbreviated history of medicine and how it evolved into the overcomplicated, complex system of healing that is practiced today. From this condensed retelling of events, one can glean that the process of 'curing' disease does not have to be the expensive and often invasive procedure it presently is. There is an easier, more organic and far more effective approach to curing disease and maintaining good health—one that has been obscured by the highly complex science (and business) of medicine and pharmaceuticals.

Ever since the dawn of medicine centuries ago, misinformation about healing has been propagated to the public through various methods. The earliest method used, especially during the Black Death in the 14th and 15th centuries, was the 'traditional authority' approach to science and medicine. This consisted of the idea that if a prominent person declared something to be true, then it must be so—and anything observed to the contrary was regarded as an anomaly.

Centuries later, physicians like Ibn al-Nafis (regarded as 'the greatest physiologist of the Middle Ages') and Vesalius (founder of modern human anatomy) replaced previous doctrines and discredited many of the theories of 'traditional authorities' with doctrines derived from their explorations in physiology and anatomy.

Fast forward to the 20th century—evidence-based medicine began to emerge, wherein the most effective ways of doing things (also called 'algorithms of practice' or 'best practice') were identified through scientific methods and modern global information science. The evidence was collated; standard protocols were developed, and thereafter disseminated to doctors and healthcare providers. The problem with the 'best practice' approach is that it served to suppress all other alternative approaches to treatment.

Furthermore, the scientific methods used in drawing conclusions, although seemingly logical and unbiased (therefore, reliable), were actually *flawed.*

All scientific experimentation is subject to *confirmation* bias (or the *observer-expectancy effect*) to a certain extent. Confirmation bias is an unfair influence found in scientific research when a researcher expects a given result, and therefore, *unconsciously* manipulates an experiment in order to find that result. A researcher's particular ideology, worldview, superstitions, traditions or religion can cause him or her to assign greater weight to some data over other data. The human brain has a tendency to fill in the gaps of what it perceives, and oftentimes, a researcher may also be stubborn, unwilling to admit a mistake, or embarrassed by having to withdraw a publicly declared belief. Thus, any conclusions derived from "scientific studies" or "clinical studies" are rarely unbiased, and thus, cannot always be regarded as reliable.

At present, there exists a confusing array of so-called 'best practices' for every part of the anatomy, all *tainted with bias* to one degree or another. This has made the curing of diseases *seem* like a complex and mysterious science with its own language that is beyond the understanding of the non-medical population—like the scriptural Tower of Babel that brought about a confusion of tongues.

What complicates the matter is that the field of medicine has given rise to a slew of organ-based specializations such as neurology, cardiology, dermatology, ophthalmology, urology, gynecology, endocrinology, etc.—as well as disease-based specializations such as oncology (for cancer), gerontology (for diseases of the aging) that each have their respective modes of treatment and therapy. The end result is a medical model not unlike the legend from India about the 6 blind men who encountered an elephant.

The Legend of the
6 Blind Men and the Elephant

There once were 6 blind men who, upon encountering an elephant, gave their own individual assessments of the elephant. The first one happened to fall against the broad and sturdy side of the elephant, and concluded that the elephant is very much like a *wall*. The second one, feeling the tusk, said the elephant was very much like a *spear*. The third one happened to take the squirming trunk in his hands, and said the elephant was very much like a *snake*. The fourth one, reached out and touched the elephant's knee, and concluded that the elephant is very much like a *tree*. The fifth one happened to touch the ear, and insisted that the elephant is very much like a *fan*. And the sixth one seized the swinging tail, and said the elephant is very much like a *rope*.

Each of the blind men was partly right based on his own subjective perception—but at the same time, *mostly wrong*. The comical part of it all is that their dispute stemmed from utter ignorance because none had ever seen the elephant!

The field of medicine, with its compartmentalized theories about what causes disease and how to eradicate it from the human body, actually perceives only a *small snapshot* of the larger picture, a *localized subset* of the larger workings of the human body.

One would think that because the medical and pharmaceutical industries have grown as large as they have, that we would have less sick people in the world. But the opposite is actually true. There are more sick people in the U.S., for instance, than at any other time in history—not just in actual numbers but as a percentage of the population.

This, in no way, is intended to discredit doctors, medical practitioners and institutions that have genuinely good intentions of helping to heal people and eradicate disease. It simply points to an ineffective medical system that is focused on illness rather than wellness, that promotes expensive (i.e., profit-driven), invasive and potentially dangerous (or even deadly) medical procedures, drugs or treatments rather than simple, natural, inexpensive, effective treatments or therapies that have no side effects.

There's a Chinese proverb which says:

The *superior* doctor prevents illness.
The *mediocre* doctor attends to impending sickness.
The *inferior doctor* treats actual illness.

According to the above definition, traditional (allopathic) doctors are either mediocre or inferior! However, they are so, not necessarily because of their mediocre or inferior dedication to the healing profession, but because all 160 medical schools that provide conventional medical education and training focus on treating actual or impending diseases rather than preventing them.

While the majority of drugs prescribed by doctors may seem to provide relief (or so-called "cure") for a **disease, most of them simply relieve symptoms or the pain associated with the disease, but <u>don't</u> actually cure the disease.** For example, the most popular asthma medications (consisting of inhaled beta-agonists), which relax airway muscles, may help asthma sufferers to breathe easier, but they do NOT cure the condition nor reduce the inflammation in the airways. The drugs that do claim to "cure" an illness by halting the spread of invading germs, such as bacteria and viruses; and by killing cells as they divide or preventing them from multiplying; do so but <u>not without harming the body to some extent.</u>

Practically **all drugs have side effects:** that is, they cause **effects** (including adverse and serious effects) other than those that are desired. Sometimes, drugs provide relief for one health problem, but in the process, give rise to even more serious health problems. So we take drugs that relieve the symptoms of osteoporosis and in turn, acquire a high risk of breast cancer; and we trade impotence for heart disease; or depression for diabetes; and take a pill for arthritis at the risk of getting a heart attack. There are even drugs that are designed primarily to alleviate the side effects caused by other drugs or medical treatments.

DID YOU KNOW THAT... properly administered prescription drugs **kill** over 100,000 people per year? Not mistakes. Not overdoses. "Properly prescribed" medications given to people in hospitals are toxic enough to kill over 100,000 people per year.

Source: "Incidence of Adverse Drug Reactions in Hospitalized Patients", Journal of the American Medical Association

(This statistic did NOT count all the deaths that occurred due to drugs if the problem occurred at the person's home.)

The foregoing is only in reference to the side effects of *drugs*. There are also side effects and serious health consequences that come with medical treatments like surgery, radiation or chemotherapy, for example. And even diagnostic procedures like X-Rays, mammograms and MRIs have their own attendant risks and side effects.

Case in Point: Ever since mammograms were introduced, the incidence of ductal carcinoma in situ (DCIS), a **type of breast cancer, has increased by 328%!** At least 200% of this increase is attributed to the harmful radiation of mammograms. Furthermore, mammograms are also thought to help spread existing cancer cells due to the considerable pressure placed on the breast during the procedure.

When you consider the prevailing conditions that exist in the medical industry, you begin to see that your best interests are not served by relinquishing total control of your health to doctors, medical establishments or the pharmaceutical industry.

What this means to you is that you must not blindly accept medical advice as the best course of action for your health. Neither should you be deceived by the multi-million dollar advertising campaigns of the pharmaceutical companies that promote **"medicines" that do not cure and often harm.**

The Most Essential Element in the Human Body

In order to dismantle the complex healing modalities that the medical and pharmaceutical industries have created—and discover the path to true healing—one needs to take a closer look at the core of human existence. The human body is composed of 70%-80% water—and water is 89% oxygen by weight. Therefore, **oxygen comprises 62% to 71% of the body,** and is the body's most abundant and essential element.

Ninety (90%) percent of all our biological energy comes from oxygen. It is the essential element that the human body needs in order to not only survive, but also have optimum levels of energy, function properly and become more productive.

Consider, for instance, that humans can survive for weeks and even months without food, and live for many days without water. But we cannot survive more than a few minutes without oxygen.

Most people overlook the fact that the very element—which is required by all humans in order to live—is also the **secret** to keeping us disease-free. Medical professionals, in particular, would find the notion of curing virtually all diseases with oxygen rather simplistic, or even lacking merit.

The curious thing is that oxygen is already used in medicine. Oxygen supplementation has been used to ease health conditions, such as emphysema and pneumonia that impair the body's ability to have a sufficient intake of gaseous oxygen. Hyperbaric (high-pressure) oxygen has been used to treat carbon monoxide poisoning, gas gangrene and decompression sickness. Oxygen has also been used for life support situations and on patients who require mechanical ventilation. Patients on their deathbed who are given extra doses of oxygen are often kept alive long after they would otherwise have died.

However, because oxygen has seldom been used in the medical setting as a *first line of defense* for preventing, let alone "curing" diseases, it has never been accorded its rightful place as the cure for virtually all diseases.

The world of science and medicine has always known that oxygen is the basis of human life, without which humans die. This fundamental truth has become so overlaid with centuries' worth of extraneous matter that its essence has become completely obscured by the 'Tower of Babel' created by the field of medicine.

This book will provide solid proof that the **primary physical cause of all diseases** is linked in one way or another to *oxygen deficiency.* In fact, many of the elaborate (and expensive) therapies offered by organized medicine take advantage of oxygen's effect on diseased cells. Most conventional cancer therapies, for instance, including chemotherapy and radiation therapy, produce oxygen-activated events that kill cancer cells. A cancer drug named verteporfin, increases the amount of oxygen within cancerous tumors, and this kills tumors more effectively than radiation alone. Interferon drugs, which are vastly prescribed for the treatment of multiple sclerosis, owe their efficacy to the fact that they raise the body's oxygen level. One could draw the conclusion that many drugs basically work on the same principle of oxygenation described in this book, but those drugs cost tens of thousands times more than the pennies-a-day self-administered therapy I present herein. Furthermore, the therapy I present does not come with any of the adverse effects typically associated with toxic drugs and other radical medical therapies.

In the following chapters, you will discover ...

- how dozens of AIDS patients have reversed their death sentences and are now living normal lives as a result of this little-known therapy involving oxygen;

- how all disease-causing microorganisms, viruses (including coronavirus), harmful bacteria, toxins and pathogens are eradicated in the presence of sufficient amounts of oxygen in the blood and cells;

- how a great number of diseases ranging from colds and the common flu to malaria and cholera have been cured as far back as 180 years ago in India using this same therapy;

- why the handful of U.S. doctors who employ this therapy to cure a wide variety of so-called "incurable" diseases, or endorse the therapy in any way, come under heavy attack by the medical establishment and are threatened with the revocation of their medical licenses; and

- how you can oxygenate your body using a remarkably simple procedure without the aid of a doctor—and duplicate the spectacular healing results of institutional oxygen therapy at home in one minute or less.

Although the fundamental concept behind the one-minute oxygen therapy is based on a centuries-old truth, it has just been rediscovered and repurposed for use in today's world. As with any newly discovered truth, it must necessarily pass through 3 stages: First, it is ridiculed. Then, it is violently opposed. Finally, it is accepted as self-evident.

The truth contained in this book is already self-evident to people in many parts of the world. Many people have awakened to the realization that a simple at-home procedure involving an oxygenating substance represents the "cutting edge" of a new healing paradigm. As more people discover this safe, effective, natural and low-cost healing modality for treating both minor health problems as well as the most devastating diseases facing mankind today—including AIDS, cancer, heart disease, Alzheimer's and Parkinson's disease—it may not only improve the quality of people's lives but also help to solve our national health care crisis.

I've written this book in hopes that this therapy will become accepted by more doctors not only in the U.S. but all over the world, and that it will become a valuable part of mainstream medical practice. It is also my vision that more people will take control of their own health and healing by using this therapy, and that we will finally have a world free of virtually all diseases.

~ CHAPTER TWO ~

In this chapter, I will reveal the secret to oxygenating your body in a way that will ward off disease, and in case you have already acquired a disease, give you an easy way to get rid of it. The oxygen therapy presented herein does not actually "cure" disease, but rather creates an environment in your body that is uninhabitable by disease microorganisms, viruses, harmful bacteria and pathogens. Therefore, you'll effectively be enabling your body to *heal itself.*

Disease is Big Business: The Awful Truth

FACT: Americans spend more on health care, yet are sicker than most other people in the world. Americans suffer from higher incidences of cancer, heart disease, diabetes, rheumatoid arthritis, lung disease and a host of other diseases—even though all those diseases are both *preventable* and *curable.*

It's a sad fact that despite massive expenditures on medical treatments and drugs, Americans are sicker than ever before in our history. One might wonder why the so-called "miracle drugs" manufactured and promoted by pharmaceutical companies—not to mention the highly touted medical "breakthroughs"—have neither prevented nor cured disease in this country and the world.

The answer is this: **Disease is big business.**

In 2019, before the pandemic, Americans spent $3.8

trillion on health care, according to HealthSystemTracker. org. This translates to $11,582 per person. Approximately half of the spending is on **pharmaceutical drugs.**

With these kinds of revenues, there is no incentive on the part of the pharmaceutical industries to promote better health. They are the most profitable industry in the world, enjoying average profit margins of 30,000% to 50,000% on pharmaceutical drugs over the cost of raw materials. Sometimes, their markups can be as high as 569,000%! The average business person in his right mind wouldn't dare walk away from such profits, and would do almost anything to ensure that the trillion-dollar cash cow remains intact.

As a result, the pharmaceutical industry has assembled a pharma-cartel consisting of an army of lobbyists that influence not only the entire medical industry but also the U.S. Congress; and by extension, the lives of the entire American population. Pharmaceutical companies spend enormous amounts of money to get doctors to prescribe their drugs to patients; to get the American public to believe, via the barrage of drug commercials, that they've got a health problem; and to get Congress to pass legislation that ensures their continued profitability.

Case in Point: An investigative report, which aired on the popular CBS program, *Sixty Minutes,* revealed that "Congressmen are outnumbered 2 to 1 by lobbyists for the pharmaceutical industry that spends roughly $100 million a year in campaign contributions and lobbying expenses to protect its profits." Because of this, the pharmaceutical lobby *almost never loses a political battle* that affects its bottom line.

In fact, there have been thousands of bills placed in front of the House of Representatives over the years dealing with pharmaceutical issues—and the drug companies, almost without exception, have gotten what they wanted.

The pharmaceutical industry has more to gain when people are sick than when they are well. Therefore, they manufacture drugs that only relieve symptoms but do not cure disease. There's a vested interest in keeping people sick because the big bucks are in drugs for ongoing diseases. And yet, the pharmaceutical companies' clever propaganda to make themselves look like the savior of all mankind—a savior that finds "cures" for diseases and saves people's lives—has successfully deceived us into regarding them with a sense of awe, reverence and respect for all that they do for human health.

The irony of it all is that **more people have died from preventable diseases than all the wars of the world combined** as a direct result of the pharmaceutical business. These deaths were not just from the use of drugs but from the industry's **suppression of information about non-drug health alternatives** that could have kept people from dying.

Pharmaceutical companies routinely use their power and unlimited financial resources to keep doctors from prescribing natural therapies—and their powerful lobbyists even get Congress to **disallow established health claims for natural remedies.** If you conduct some research on your own, you'll find this to be true. They have built an elaborate maze of manipulation, control, infiltration and economic incentives to systematically deceive millions of people into thinking that drugs are the only solution to disease.

The deception has become so pervasive that we have been brainwashed into thinking that whenever we are sick or are not feeling well, all we have to do is take a pill to feel better. The truth is, no matter how much the drug companies want you to believe that it's "normal" to take medicine every day (or multiple drugs a day, in some instances), it's not. In the words of one world-renowned doctor who's been recently silenced for speaking the truth, **"It is the rare exception that you should ever need to take a drug."**

It is of no comfort that the Food & Drug Administration (FDA), the government agency created to protect public health, makes it a priority to promote drugs and the financial interests of pharmaceutical companies. This is so because many of the FDA's senior management and members of its advisory committees accept more than $50,000 apiece in corporate grants, contracts and consulting fees from pharmaceutical companies. It wasn't until the Vioxx scandal took place that the true nature of the FDA was revealed, along with its leniency toward the industry it's supposed to be regulating. In 2004, Merck marketed Vioxx for the treatment of arthritis and other conditions causing chronic or acute pain. Later, it was discovered that Merck had deliberately suppressed the heart attack risks of Vioxx. The international medical community has criticized the FDA for not only being "asleep at the wheel" while this was happening, but also of acting in collusion with Merck to cover up the truth. The irresponsible behavior of the FDA caused Dr. Richard Horton, editor of *The Lancet* (one of the most respected medical journals in the world) to state, "This discovery points to astonishing failures in Merck's internal systems of post-marketing surveillance, as well as to **lethal weaknesses** in the U.S. Food and Drug Administration's regulatory oversight." Vioxx has since been taken off the market.

Fictitious Diseases Abound

Those in the wholistic health field have known for a long time that fictitious diseases are "invented" all the time by the pharmaceutical industry for no reason other than to sell prescription drugs. If you've ever wondered why all of a sudden, there's an entire array of new diseases that were unheard of 20 years ago or more, this is the reason. Diseases like *intermittent explosive disorder (bad temper), bereavement-associated depression (grief), hypoactive sexual disorder* (low sex drive), pornography addiction, compulsive buying or gambling, excessive Internet use, ADD (attention deficit disorder) and ADHD (attention deficit hyperactivity disorder) are examples of such so-called diseases.

ADD and ADHD, for instance, are simply conditions usually brought about by the overconsumption of refined sugar, junk food and soft drinks by children. The media declares ADHD an 'epidemic' of sorts because there are reportedly 6.1 million children in America (13% of the country's schoolchildren) who are diagnosed with ADHD, according to the Centers for Disease Control (CDC) website. The drug, Ritalin, became so popular because they made ADHD a bonafide disease that required a prescription. And psychiatrists were only too happy because they got kickbacks from drug companies every time they prescribed Ritalin for kids who really were just a bit overactive (probably because of their overconsumption of sugar).

Furthermore, in recent years, there has been an upsurge in the use of powerful psychotropic, mind-altering drugs to children as young as 2 and 3 years old (at least in foster homes) because it is much cheaper and easier to keep them quiet than providing time-consuming care. The number of prescriptions for "chemical straightjacket" drugs like Prozac, Paxil, Zyprexa and Depakote has more than doubled in the last 16 years.

Clearly, the pharmaceutical industry wants to categorize the majority of the population as having some kind of disorder. And if there isn't a legitimate disorder, why, one can always be invented! *Social anxiety disorder* (shyness or lack of social skills) and fear of public speaking are just two so-called disorders that attempt to encompass the entire population. Everyone suffers from one degree of shyness or another, depending on the social situation, and fear of public speaking is a natural fear that most people have. These are not diseases at all, but rather normal human tendencies or behavioral differences. But when they're categorized as disorders, doctors are given the freedom to "push" a variety of drugs on you—such as duloxetine for bereavement, escitalopram for excessive Internet use, divalproex sodium for intermittent explosive disorder, topiramate for compulsive gambling, fluvoxamine for compulsive buying, naltrexone for pornography addiction, and quetiapine for fear of public speaking.

The *Physicians Desk Reference* (PDR) is considered the

medical bible of drugs, wherein all prescription drugs are compiled (and which is updated annually) for use by doctors in prescribing drugs. If you look up a prescription drug in the PDR, you'll find its "mechanism of action," which is the mechanism by which the drug produces an effect on a living organism or in a biochemical system. Frequently, the mechanism of action for a great number of drugs is listed as "unknown." Sometimes the mechanism of action is stated in phrases such as "it *appears* to be" or "it is thought to" or "it is believed that" which are not scientific words, but rather words that suggest educated guesses rather than information based on concrete scientific evidence.

For example, almost all psychotropics (i.e., drugs used in the treatment of mental illnesses) have an unknown mechanism of action, and yet they're wantonly prescribed because they've "been demonstrated to" quiet down lab monkeys and prisoners. Statins are another class of drugs that have an unknown mechanism of action, and yet doctors prescribe them like candy even though they cause a wide array of adverse effects ranging from statin-induced myopathy (progressive weakness of the muscles) to cytotoxic effects to testicular pain. Additionally, once you begin a statin regimen, you usually have to take the statin for life or you run the risk of getting a heart attack, which is what happened to former Vice President Al Gore after he stopped taking statins.

It bears repeating that most prescription drugs are unnecessary, and that they could actually be "killing you legally" not to mention *robbing you blind.* Instead of relying on drugs and contributing to the $1.3 trillion dollar revenues of Big Pharma (Source: Statista.com) for drugs that do not cure— and often cause harm, or even death—we must rely more on natural approaches for achieving optimal health.

Nutrition is Big Business, Too

I've been both an aficionado and avid researcher of natural and wholistic approaches to health since 1978, and have also written articles about them as a contributing editor for wholistic health publications. As such, I've witnessed an endless parade of "natural" remedies and therapies go by in the last 40 years—some having merit and others providing little or no health benefit at all.

I've also seen countless products with marginal health benefits masquerading as 'breakthrough' discoveries when in actuality, they're nothing more than marketing puffery and shrewd advertising designed to capitalize on health trends. Oftentimes, I've observed hundreds, or even thousands of business enterprises spring up out of nowhere to cash in on such trends and fads.

Case in Point: The popularity of *Dead Doctors Don't Lie,* an audio presentation by veterinarian and naturopath Dr. Joel Wallach explaining his core ideas about health and nutrition, sparked the frenzy over colloidal minerals in the 1990s. In the audiotape, which was reportedly distributed to over 50 million people, Dr. Wallach asserted that: 1) mineral deficiencies are responsible for most chronic diseases; and 2) only minerals in "colloidal" form contain all the essential minerals that can be adequately absorbed by the human body.

As a result of that audiotape, a proliferation of expensive colloidal mineral supplements flooded the market and stocked the shelves of health food stores everywhere— even though no peer-reviewed scientific work has shown colloidal minerals to have any more absorbability than normal minerals, and the health claims were anecdotal and scientifically unproven.

The above example shows how the antiquated 'traditional authority' approach to science and medicine used in the 15th and 16th century is alive and well in the modern world. The 'traditional authority' approach, as discussed in the previous chapter, consists of the idea that if a prominent person declares something to be true, then it must be so. In today's society, however, it doesn't even require a prominent person to establish something as the truth. Sometimes, all it takes is a charismatic speaker who has the ability to make a credible argument, or a brilliant marketer that can capture the imagination of the buying public and build an enormous marketing empire from a small morsel of information that isn't even an established fact.

For as long as the natural health and wellness movement has been in existence, health fads and trends that were founded on misinformation or erroneous factoids have come and gone. Following are just a few of them:

- The popularity of margarine and hydrogenated oils as a "healthier" substitute for butter and animal fats started in the late 1950s and early 1960s when it was thought that there was a correlation between heart disease and animal fat consumption. This was disproven in 2000 when it was discovered that trans-fatty acids, which are present in chemically hydrogenated oils and margarine, have harmful effects that are even worse than the consumption of animal fat. Trans-fats have been linked to increased rates of coronary heart disease and cancer, as well as other chronic diseases.

- Millions of Americans have been taking high doses of beta carotene because it was initially thought to prevent cancer and heart disease. This has since been disproven by several multiple-year studies, including one involving 18,000 subjects that showed no significant reduction in heart disease—and actually **29% more incidences of lung cancer**—than those who received a placebo. It turns out that the initial observational studies of large populations showing that people who eat a lot of beta-carotene-rich fruits and vegetables tended to have a low risk of cancer, heart disease and heart attacks did not necessarily mean that beta carotene supplementation would be just as effective.

- Over the last several decades, supplement manufacturers (and even health practitioners) have urged people to take large amounts of antioxidants such as Vitamin C, Vitamin E, super oxide dismutase (SOD), because such nutritional supplements supposedly scavenge free radicals which cause cell damage. However, it has since been demonstrated in the laboratory that dosing a culture of cells with these antioxidants does not decrease free radical production by any significant amount. It has also been shown that when a person swallows antioxidants, the digestive juices *nullify* any free radical scavenging action long before the antioxidants come in contact with the cells they are meant to protect.

- Gelatin capsules have long been touted as being the best thing one can do to strengthen fingernails. While gelatin does contain collagen, which is a protein found in nails and other body tissues, it has been disproven that gelatin supplementation has any fingernail-building benefits at all.

- In 1986, canola oil was touted as being a healthy oil because it is lower in saturated fat (6%) than any other oil. In contrast, peanut oil contains 18%, and palm oil, 79%. Because canola oil also contains cholesterol-balancing monounsaturated fat comparable to olive oil, the Canola Council of Canada attempted to link many of the benefits of olive oil-rich Mediterranean-type diets to diets high in canola oil—even if canola oil has never been used in Mediterranean cuisine. The propaganda worked, and sales of canola oil have been on the upswing ever since. However, not too many people know that frying with canola oil releases toxic, carcinogenic fumes. In at least 2 studies, it was shown that high lung cancer rates in Chinese women were linked to wok cooking with canola (also called rapeseed) oil. Consumption of canola oil has been shown to cause fibrotic lesions of the heart, CNS degenerative disorders, prostate cancer, anemia, lung cancer, constipation, irritation of the mucous membranes and many toxic effects, according to many nutritionists and biochemists.

Why have I found it necessary to present the above abbreviated list of health fads and disproven myths about food products and nutritional supplements? It's to point out 3 important factors you must remember in the quest for health and the prevention/cure of disease:

Nutrition is big business, too. According to *Nutrition Business Journal* (NBJ), the estimated size of the U.S. global nutrition industry is $140 billion. While many companies in the nutrition marketplace are upstanding enterprises that conduct their businesses ethically, their lifeblood still depends on how creatively they market their products to differentiate them from their competitors.

Considering the abundance of unsubstantiated health claims and hoaxes that exist in the nutrition marketplace, it would serve your best interests to be wary of how profit-driven companies will use the power of enticing *pseudo-logic* and *double-speak* (supported by emotional appeals to your fear of disease) to sell you their products. Some creative marketers will even resort to instilling the belief in you that "scientists" know more about health than you do. They will reinforce your need for their products through exposure to advertisements and propaganda that most people cannot resist.

Companies that have a common interest in promoting and protecting the financial interests of specific industries often form organizations or associations that do cooperative advertising and promotions for their respective industries. These are all meant to shape the public's perception of the products they sell. The American Egg Board, for instance, came up with the "incredible edible egg™" campaign and positioned eggs as nature's miracle food to counteract the mounting criticism that eggs are the major culprit in the nation's high cholesterol problem. Likewise, the Canola Council of Canada not only renamed the rapeseed oil to the mellifluous-sounding "canola" oil but also positioned it as a healthy oil compared to other vegetable oils.

Any food product or nutritional supplement can be made to appear like a miracle cure or an essential health-enhancing or disease-preventing product that no one can live without—as long as it is marketed properly. An advertiser can make a product seem to have **curative** properties —while still staying within the advertising restrictions established by the Federal Trade Commission (FTC) and the FDA—by using terminology similar to that used by pharmaceutical companies when their drug's mechanism of action is unknown. Phrases such as "it *appears* to be" or "it is thought to" or "it is *believed* that" are used liberally, as well as phrases like "this has been shown to" and "this helps to" or "this assists in."

One important guideline to follow is that whenever you come across information about a food product or nutritional supplement, which is disseminated by a company or organization that sells that food product or nutritional supplement—or stands to gain financially from the dissemination of the information—consider the information skewed to their favor and therefore, unreliable. Instead, seek out products recognized by third-party experts who are able to filter through the marketing hype fabricated by health product manufacturers and distributors.

Don't jump to irrational conclusions. More often than not, people make *emotional* decisions in matters concerning their health rather than using rational thinking. Marketers and advertisers are aware of this, and that is why they will often appeal to your emotion in an effort to sell their products. A company might use the following emotional appeal, for instance: "Magnesium deficiency is the cause of most serious diseases" and go on to say that their magnesium supplements will take care of that deficiency. This might then cause you to draw the conclusion that they wanted you to draw in the first place, and that is to believe that taking their magnesium supplement will prevent you from getting those serious diseases. Being unaware of such marketing ploys, particularly the clever appeal to your fear of disease, could cause you to make irrational decisions without first investigating the validity of their claims.

Consider the big picture. One thing that the above examples indicate is the fact that the field of natural health and nutrition—just like the field of medicine—has developed its own compartmentalized theories about what causes disease, and how to prevent and heal it. Therefore, focus is oftentimes placed on only a *small snapshot* of the larger picture—a *localized subset* of the larger workings of the human body.

The point is, there now exist a multitude of so-called "natural" approaches to disease prevention and treatment. Unfortunately, most of them offer a myopic, incomplete view of the whole human organism—not unlike the blind men making individual assessments about the elephant, and none of them quite hitting the mark!

If you happen to be a health-conscious individual, take a look at the nutritional supplements you take. How many are you taking on a regular basis? How much are they costing you? Which of them are really good for your health—and which aren't? Which of them will prevent you from getting cancer or any other disease—or cure you if you already have the disease? These are the kinds of questions I've asked myself throughout the 40 years that I've been researching natural approaches to health.

The biggest mistake I've seen people make is that they fail to see the larger picture—that is, how the whole human organism works, as well as the interactions of the different elements in the human body. One should always be aware that a considerable number of so-called health products often ignore the entire biochemistry of the human body.

Wonder Cure or Snake Oil?

Separating the wheat from the chaff when it comes to natural health products, differentiating health fads from bonafide health items—and trying to distinguish between commercial propaganda versus trustworthy information presented with no profit-driven agenda—is a daunting task for anyone. This is true particularly because a wide assortment of so-called nutritional breakthroughs (or super foods) fall in and out of grace, and dozens more arrive at the scene almost every day. Oftentimes, one rarely knows which of them really work and which ones are the products of clever marketing.

It was while I was keeping abreast of the continuously expanding—and overwhelming!—array of products and services in the natural health field that I came across a piece of information about oxygen therapy that was positively **astounding**. Since I had known about oxygen therapy for decades, and had even written about it on a few occasions, I was tempted to dismiss the information or conclude that I knew all about it already. I'm glad that, instead, I chose to give it the renewed attention it deserved.

I remember when I first heard about this little-known aspect of oxygen therapy (which involves hydrogen peroxide), my heart pounded with excitement, realizing that this may be the closest thing to a panacea that the world has ever known. As I expanded my research, I was dumbfounded by the mountains of evidence showing that hydrogen peroxide therapy has been used in various parts of the world by over 15,000 European doctors, naturopaths and homeopaths. Its use goes as far back as 180 years ago, and has healed millions of patients of almost every disease known to man, including "the big 3"—AIDS, cancer and heart disease. I began wondering why I hadn't encountered this information before, and more importantly, why the whole world didn't already know about this. I soon realized why.

This simple, effective and inexpensive therapy for eradicating disease threatens the trillion-dollar pharmaceutical cartel. As discussed in the previous chapter, when *anything* threatens the bottom line profits of the pharmaceutical industry, it will be suppressed, lobbied against or given a negative spin so as to ridicule it, outlaw it and render it worthless. Additionally, individuals who perpetrate the perceived threat are often imprisoned, their businesses (or practices, in the case of health practitioners) shut down, or forbidden from dispensing health advice again.

In my view, however, the hydrogen peroxide therapy I reveal in this book is far too valuable to human health to keep under wraps. I'm able to write about it only because I have a disclaimer in the beginning of the book that says the information contained herein is for educational purposes only and not meant to diagnose illness or meant to replace a doctor's advice.

Even as I write this, I realize that initiatives may already be in place to take food-grade hydrogen peroxide out of the market because it presents a threat to the revenues of the pharmaceutical industry. The pharmaceutical companies are looking for legitimate ways to discredit food-grade hydrogen peroxide and call it hazardous—or even poisonous— even though hydrogen peroxide has been given the GRAS designation (Generally Recognized as Safe) by the FDA.

My stand on this matter is that it would be downright criminal not to disseminate information about the therapeutic benefits of food-grade hydrogen oxygen—especially since its dissemination could not only potentially save people's lives, but also improve the quality of their lives.

The reasons why the therapeutic use of food-grade hydrogen peroxide is the most exciting therapy to come around in the health and healing horizon are *seven-fold:*

1 Therapeutic use of food-grade hydrogen peroxide is a systemic therapy (i.e., affecting the body as a *whole*, rather than one specific organ or part). Thus, it **creates an environment in the body that enables the body to cure itself** of virtually all diseases caused by viruses, harmful bacteria, toxins, disease microorganisms and pathogens, including—but not limited to—cancer, AIDS, Alzheimer's and Parkinson's Disease, diabetes, rheumatoid arthritis, multiple sclerosis, heart disease, ulcers, asthma and many other types of diseases, including the flu.

2 Unlike other so-called "cures" that tend to get inordinately focused on small details of biochemistry, oxygen therapy via food-grade hydrogen peroxide is predicated on providing the most abundant and essential element of the human body. The body may need an array of different elements and nutrients such as CoQ10, magnesium, Omega-3 fatty acids and the like, but only oxygen is in such critical demand that an insufficient supply makes the body develop diseases, and its absence causes the body to die within minutes. Oxygen is what makes life possible, and therefore, it's a virtual *infusion of "life force."*

3 Literature that proclaim the so-called healing benefits of other health and nutrition products are usually compiled by people who stand to gain financially from the sale of those products (which usually have very high profit margins). Therefore, the accuracy and reliability of such information is suspect. In contrast, the information contained in this book (along with science-backed literature you might find regarding the therapeutic benefits of food-grade hydrogen peroxide) is **not motivated by profiteering.** Food-grade hydrogen peroxide is a chemical that cannot be patented, has a very low profit margin, and is widely available—therefore making it unlikely to be overpriced by profiteers. Food-grade hydrogen peroxide **costs only 1½ cents a day** for the recommended dosage, and takes **less than one minute** to administer. Others claim to have developed machines that produce oxygen-saturated water, which supposedly provides a rich source of extra oxygen in a highly absorbable form—but you'll end up paying a small fortune (up to $3,980) and at best, get the same benefits you'd get for pennies by using food-grade hydrogen peroxide.

4 Unlike other cures that may only be applicable to a certain segment of the population, oxygen therapy via food-grade hydrogen peroxide has universal application in humans (with the exception of people who have organ transplants). It can even be used with pets.

5 Conventional therapies usually harm good cells in the body in the process of "curing" disease. Pharmaceutical drugs and medical treatments—such as chemotherapy—are examples of such therapies which not only harm good cells but also shut down the body's immune system at a time when the body needs it most. The use of food-grade hydrogen peroxide, on the other hand, creates an environment in the body that **kills viruses, harmful bacteria, toxins, pathogens and disease microorganisms while contributing to the vitality of healthy cells.** Because of the increased oxygen supply brought about by hydrogen peroxide, the immune system is also boosted, thereby enabling the body to ward off disease and heal itself.

6 Many so-called "cures" are often just another player in a long line of health fads. After having witnessed many such fads being hailed as the "be-all end-all" cure, only to be disproven by the next latest study (also motivated by financial gain), I've decided to put credence only on those **therapies that have stood the test of time.** Successful therapeutic use of hydrogen peroxide goes back over 180 years ago, and is validated by 91,000 scientific studies, even though its use is largely suppressed in the U.S.

7 Using healing therapies based on scientific evidence that encompass only a small aspect of the human body's biochemistry is like cooking in the dark. You're likely to get undesirable side effects (e.g., when you take mega-doses of Vitamin C, you could unduly tax your liver; or when you consume colloidal silver for a prolonged period of time, you could develop blue skin pigmentation). Oxygen therapy, on the other hand, takes into consideration **the human body's chemical constituents and their interaction with each other within the biochemical parameters of the body.** As long as hydrogen peroxide is diluted in distilled water in the recommended concentration, and taken on an empty stomach (see Chapter 5 for correct administration), its **disease-fighting constituents are maximized and adverse effects become virtually non-existent**

~ CHAPTER THREE ~

The Most Dreaded Diseases of All Time

What diseases do people fear the most? Depending on which survey you rely on, you may discover that the following are invariably the 5 most dreaded diseases of all time:

Cancer
Heart Disease
Stroke
Diabetes
Alzheimer's Disease

There are officially more than 12,420 documented diseases in the world, according to the World Health Organization (WHO).

It's not surprising that AIDS also ranks as one of the top 10 most feared diseases—for many reasons: Almost everyone is susceptible to the deadly disease; the number of people diagnosed with AIDS in the U.S. has multiplied by a factor of 34 since 2008 (source: Centers for Disease Control); and most importantly, AIDS is regarded as not only **incurable, but also fatal.**

How would your fear of AIDS be tempered if you knew that dozens of AIDS patients have **not only reversed their death sentences, but have become completely free of the disease** and now live normal, healthy lives? (See page 49)

No discussion of dreaded diseases would be complete without mentioning COVID-19, which is in a category all by itself as *the most feared viral disease*. However, once you understand its true underpinnings, you'll be able to put your fear of COVID-19 in context. (See page 89)

Now, let's consider the most dreaded disease in America and the world, "the big C"—*cancer*. The 3 words a doctor can say that strikes the most fear in people are: "You've got cancer." Every 3 minutes, someone new is diagnosed with cancer—and cancer is among the leading causes of death worldwide. There's practically no one in America who does not personally know someone who has been diagnosed with—or has died of—cancer. **Approximately 39.5% of men and women will be diagnosed with cancer at some point during their lifetimes** *(Source: cancer.gov),* and an estimated 560,000 Americans will die from cancer each year (roughly 1,534 deaths per day).

This forecast seems quite terrifying, to say the least. But what if I told you that there is a remarkable therapy that routinely **"cures"** cancer—even in cases when the disease wasn't caught early—and even if it happened to be late-stage terminal cancer? Would you believe that this is possible— and that these kinds of cures are already happening every day around the world?

I was initially skeptical when I first encountered the simple therapy that reportedly brought about these miraculous cures. However, the results of the countless case studies were so conclusive, and the evidence so irrefutable that I was soon convinced without a doubt that this was mankind's absolute best weapon for preventing and healing not just the most dreaded diseases—but virtually all diseases.

If you or your loved ones are suffering from any disease that is characterized by viruses, harmful bacteria, toxins, pathogens and other disease microorganisms, you cannot afford to be without the therapy described in this book. Or if you happen to be one of the countless people who fears that one day you'll get a disease that "runs in the family" or maybe develop one of many diseases that comes from getting older or from bad lifestyle choices, this therapy will lay your fears to rest.

What is Oxygen Therapy?

Oxygen therapy is a term that refers to a number of different practices in which oxygen, ozone or hydrogen peroxide are administered for therapeutic purposes. While there are various forms of oxygen therapy, much of the discussion in this book will focus on the therapeutic use of **medical ozone** and **hydrogen peroxide** (also called **bio-oxidative therapies**), which have yielded the most stunning effects in reversing the broadest spectrum of diseases.

More and more people around the world are regarding these tandem therapies as a cure-all for a variety of diseases and ailments, and they are fast becoming the methods of choice for eradicating disease.

Oxygen therapy is not new. The very first recorded case in which oxygen was actually employed as a medical remedy was in 1783 by the French physician, Caillens, who treated a female patient with daily inhalations of oxygen and successfully cured her of phthisis (an archaic name for tuberculosis). The results of the therapy were published in the *Gazette de Sante*. In 1820, practical observations on the use of oxygen in the cure of diseases were published by Dr. Daniel Hill, a surgeon who was one of the early advocates of oxygen therapy. Oxygen therapy was cited as being instrumental in successfully treating cases of nervous debility, epilepsy, hydrocephalus, and scrophula.

In 1857, *The Lancet* published an article by S.B. Birch, M.D. wherein it was suggested that a diseased patient needs "more oxygen than he can possibly obtain under many circumstances and in many diseased states from the atmosphere around him." He further wrote that oxygen may well be a powerful therapeutic agent, but at the time, the medical profession overlooked or ignored oxygen as medicine due to the lack of fair trials on a sufficient scale in practice.

Throughout the rest of the 19th century, superoxigenation and inhalation of oxygen gas were recognized as having therapeutic value, and as an effective remedy in disease. The 20th century ushered in the use of oxygen in medicine and surgery, as well as intravenous injection of oxygen and oral rhythmic insufflations of oxygen for therapeutic purposes. In 1915, a German doctor named Albert Wolff became the first doctor to use ozone to treat patients with skin diseases.

In the 1950s, several German doctors began using ozone (alongside mainstream therapeutic modalities) to treat cancer. In the same decade, hyperbaric oxygen therapy started becoming the focus of many clinical trials and was used by cancer researchers. This mode of oxygen therapy employed hyperbaric chambers, wherein the patient inhales 100% oxygen at pressures greater than normal atmospheric pressure. Since the 1950s to the present, hyperbaric oxygen therapy has helped heal and restore function for people with various neurological disorders and injuries, including Alzheimer's Disease, Parkinson's Disease, diabetes, stroke, multiple sclerosis, Lou Gehrig's Disease (ALS), brain injury, learning disabilities, cerebral palsy, chronic fatigue syndrome, and autism.

Why Does Oxygen Therapy Work So Well?

As discussed in the previous chapter, **oxygen comprises 62% to 71% of the body,** and is the body's most abundant and essential element. Ninety (90%) percent of all our biological energy comes from oxygen.

Furthermore, when you consider that disease-causing microorganisms, viruses, bacteria and pathogens cannot survive in oxygen-rich environments, you begin to see why oxygen therapy is the most powerful weapon for fighting disease. A highly oxygenated body is not only immune to disease, but it also destroys disease that already exists in the body.

If oxygen were indeed a cure-all for virtually all diseases, one might jump to the erroneous conclusion that deep breathing is all one really needs to create an oxygen-rich environment in the body. Unfortunately, that isn't the case. The fact is, even if our cities, towns and other residential areas had clean air with abundant amounts of oxygen (which they don't because of air pollution), and even if human beings remembered to breathe deeply throughout the day (which they don't), it still wouldn't be possible to take in as much oxygen as our bodies need in order for healing to occur and health to be restored.

Furthermore, simply inhaling oxygen is not enough. **Only 15% of the oxygen you inhale is absorbed into the bloodstream.** Oxygen must enter the blood, and the blood, in turn, needs to deliver it to the cells and tissues of the body. This, then would raise tissue oxygen levels, kill harmful bacteria, viruses and defective tissue cells, enable healthy cells to survive and multiply more rapidly—and ultimately create a stronger immune system.

The bio-oxidative therapies presented in this book stimulate the movement of oxygen atoms from the bloodstream to the cells to a greater degree than is usually reached by other means. With higher levels of oxygen in the tissues, harmful bacteria and viruses are killed along with defective tissue cells; normal cells survive and multiply more rapidly; and the result is a healthier body.

One of the most important discoveries supporting oxygen therapy occurred in 1931, when Dr. Otto Warburg won the Nobel Prize in Physiology or Medicine for proving **that viruses cannot proliferate or exist in an environment with high levels of oxygen.** That's because viruses are anaerobic, which means that they occur and thrive in the absence of oxygen. Dr. Warburg has been quoted as saying, "Deprive a cell 35% of its oxygen for 48 hours and it may become *cancerous.*" He further stated that the prime cause of cancer is insufficient oxygen at the cellular level, and that cancer cells cannot survive in a high oxygen environment.

Risk of Getting Cancer

According to 2020 data from the American Cancer Society, men have an estimated one-in-two chance (40.14%) of developing cancer in their lifetime, with a 21.34% risk of dying from it. For women, it's slightly more than a one-in-three chance (38.7%), with an 18.33% risk of dying from it.

Additionally, <u>every human being</u> already has cancer cells proliferating in the body which are just seeking a low-oxygen environment where they can multiply into the full-blown disease.

There have been countless studies proving conclusively that increased oxygenation—whether in the form of hydrogen peroxide, ozone or hyperbaric oxygen—brings about the destruction of viruses. **Cancerous tumors shrink when put into contact with oxygen.** The studies conducted by other researchers and doctors have proven that not only cancer cells but **almost all toxins, bacteria, viruses, pathogens and disease microorganisms are oxidized and killed in high oxygen environments.** As a result, we now know that cancer and other disease-causing cells simply cannot survive and thrive in a body that is oxygen-rich. Normal cells, on the other hand, which require oxygen as their source of life, and depend on oxygen to maintain function and viability, thrive and become healthier in an oxygen-rich environment. The human body as a whole is rejuvenated and receives countless health benefits from oxygen therapy.

Louis Pasteur, the notable 19th century French chemist and microbiologist best known for his remarkable breakthroughs in the causes and prevention of disease, recanted his germ theory of disease at his deathbed, stating, "The microbe is nothing. The terrain is everything." The terrain of which he spoke is not the immune system, but the oxygenated environment of the human body. A weakened or suppressed state of the immune system only occurs when the human body lacks oxygen, thereby allowing pathogenic microbes to breed.

This was corroborated by Rudolph Virchow, the German doctor who was called the "Father of Pathology" and founded the field of Social Medicine. After an illustrious medical career, he was known to have said, "If I could live my life over again, I would devote it to proving that germs seek their natural habitat, diseased tissue, rather than being the cause of the diseased tissue; e.g., mosquitoes seek the stagnant water, but do not cause the pool to become stagnant." Likewise, **germs, bacteria, viruses and pathogens do not cause disease, but rather seek out environments where they can thrive best—and that is in oxygen-deprived bodies.**

There is now general consensus among holistic health practitioners and some enlightened members of the medical establishment about the need to oxygenate the body to prevent and even cure cancer and other degenerative diseases.

Ozone (O_3) and hydrogen peroxide (H_2O_2) are the

simplest substances available for effectively oxygenating the body. Their mechanisms of action are similar—that is, when they dissolve in the body, they both give up the extra oxygen atom in their molecular configuration, thereby producing an oxygen-rich environment in the body. Of the two substances, hydrogen peroxide is the one more readily available and easy to use.

The only reason why the medical establishment and the pharmaceutical industry haven't embraced this powerful solution for preventing and curing disease is because there is no financial incentive to do so. Both ozone and hydrogen peroxide are non-patentable substances and are very inexpensive to manufacture and use. Furthermore, as mentioned in the previous chapter, the livelihoods of doctors, hospitals and other medical establishments would be threatened if virtually all diseases were to be eradicated by the proper administration of ozone or hydrogen peroxide.

Ozone and Hydrogen Peroxide

Ozone therapy has been used with great success for a variety of diseases (see list below), including AIDS. German doctors, such as Dr. Horst Kief, Dr. S. Rilling and Dr. Renate Iffezheim have successfully treated and cured a number of AIDS patients. Several dozen AIDS patients have reversed their death sentences, thanks to the work of these doctors.

One physician from Stuttgart, Dr. Alexander Preuss, made his notes about the use of ozone therapy to treat AIDS widely available, and the results have been promising. Since Dr. Preuss made it a policy never to turn away any patients who sought ozone therapy for the treatment of AIDS, nor did he utilize any formal clinical protocol that would have rendered his findings as acceptable to the medical establishment as a clinical study, his case histories are deemed anecdotal and therefore not accepted as medical proof that the therapy is effective. However, it is undeniable that Dr. Preuss has successfully used ozone therapy to cure at least ten people of AIDS, which previously had been an incurable disease.

In the 1980s, a number of American doctors began experimenting with blood infusion of ozone to treat a variety of diseases. The Medizone Company in New York obtained permission from the FDA in 1986 to carry out experiments involving ozone therapy. The therapy involved the infusion of ozone (i.e., O_3, a "supercharged" 3-atom form of oxygen) into the blood of AIDS patients. The results were amazing. The AIDS virus was completely destroyed in vitro with no level of toxicity. The company was in the process of receiving permission from the FDA to start human testing in 1987, but the FDA suddenly stalled the process. The exact reason for the delay is unknown, but there are a variety of theories. One is that Burroughs Wellcome Company, the pharmaceutical company which had filed for a patent on AZT (the first drug for use against HIV and AIDS) in 1985, had campaigned against the Medizone human trials because AZT was about to be approved for distribution in 1987. The "official" reason given by the FDA for stalling the Medizone trials is that further testing needed to be carried out before human testing could begin. Whatever the true reason may be, the stall kept the general public unaware of the safe, effective and inexpensive treatment possibilities offered by ozone.

Unlike AIDS drugs (like AZT) which burden the liver and immune system with toxic substances, ozone overcomes the AIDS virus by simply oxidizing the molecules in the shell of the virus. When the ozone molecules dissolve into the blood, they release their 3rd oxygen atom, thereby causing hyper-oxygenation that destroys all viruses and disease microorganisms while leaving normal cells unharmed.

Today, it is possible to receive ozone therapy through blood infusions at select doctors' offices. While most traditional doctors have not yet begun offering this therapy, it is not difficult to find a list of enlightened medical practitioners, clinics and hospitals that offer ozone therapy. Just do a search on any Internet search engine, using "ozone therapy," as well as your city or country as keywords.

Blood infusion of ozone is a surprisingly simple procedure. It entails drawing a pint of blood from the patient, and introducing specific amounts of ozone into the blood through a wire cord carrying a 300- volt charge. As the ozone is absorbed by the blood, the extra oxygen atoms are released into the blood, thereby creating a flood of oxygen. The blood then turns a vivid red, which signifies healthy, oxygen-cleansed blood, and consequently, disease microorganisms are destroyed. The oxygenated blood is thereafter infused back to the patient, and as the oxygen-strengthened blood disperses, it confers some of its virucidal properties to the rest of the patient's blood, thereby destroying the diseased microorganisms in the entire body.

The procedure can be done as often as needed depending on the severity of the patient's disease. It can be used once a day, once a week, or as determined by the physician dispensing the therapy. Ozone therapy through blood infusions has been proven to successfully treat at least the following major diseases. Following is a partial list:

AIDS	Eczema
Colitis	Multiple Sclerosis
Leukemia	Acne
Alzheimer's Disease	Fungus
Cholesterol (High)	Open sores and wounds
Leg ulcers	Burns
Arteriosclerosis	Gangrene
Cystitis	Parkinson's Disease
Mononucleosis	Cancer
Arthritis	Gum disease
Proctitis	Herpes
Cardiovascular Disease	Trichomoniasis
Hepatitis	Cirrhosis of the liver
Prostate	Lymphomas
Candidiasis	Yeast & fungal infections

People have found that they remain disease-free after completion of the treatments as long as they commit to a healthier diet and exercise.

Another alternative to using ozone without the necessity of blood infusion, or without having to seek a physician who administers ozone infusion, is drinking ozonated water. Ozonated water, which is simply water that has been infused with ozone via an ozonator, is an efficient way of oxygenating the body and accelerating the healing process.

Over 100 years ago, ozone was first used to purify drinking water in Europe. Its unique characteristics make it ideally suited for water purification, and it assures you of the cleanest and safest drinking water because it eliminates 99.99% of bacteria and viruses in the water. The U.S. Environmental Protection Agency (EPA) even states that ozone is a water treatment that protects people from E-Coli.

Water ozonation is also used by various metropolitan water districts to improve the quality and taste of drinking water. Major water bottling companies utilize it for sterilization, and the food industry uses it to clean foods prior to distribution. In addition to ozone being the only natural water purification solution, research shows that **drinking ozonated water has contributed significantly to the healing of carcinoma, ulcers, gum disease, allergies, colds, flu, thrush, gastritis, cold sores, yeast infections, circulatory problems, dental infections, headaches** and a host of other ailments.

Drinking 6 to 8 glasses of ozonated water daily establishes a high level of oxygenation in the body and **accelerates the healing process.** Ozonated water also delivers the following health benefits:

- flushes toxins from your body (facilitating detoxification);

- feeds every cell with life-giving oxygen;

- sterilizes your drinking water (kills viruses, bacteria,

fungi, and algae within seconds);

- invigorates your brain and revitalizes your body all the way down to the cellular level;

- adds fuel the body needs to function; and

- makes you feel more energized and alert.

Ozonating your drinking water is quick and easy! Simply immerse the airstone (attached to your ozonator) into a glass of water and turn on the ozone generator. Ozone is thoroughly dispersed throughout the water and it's ready for drinking in a matter of minutes. To get maximum benefits, it's best to drink the water immediately after ozonating because ozone will naturally dissipate back into the surrounding air after about 20 minutes.

There are many inexpensive ozonators on the market that you can find by doing an Internet search with the key phrase "water ozonator."

While ozone administration via blood infusion or drinking ozonated water are simple protocols for fighting disease, by far the simplest, and equally viable and effective way to oxygenate the body, is via hydrogen peroxide administration. In the chapters that follow, you will learn more about discoveries surrounding the therapeutic use of hydrogen peroxide, as well as how you can use it at home to prevent and cure a wide variety of diseases and ailments.

~ CHAPTER FOUR ~

The simplest form of oxygen therapy involves the use of hydrogen peroxide because it is not only effective, but also easy enough for anyone to administer at home at a very low cost. Over the past 80 years, approximately 15,000 medical doctors, naturopaths and homeopaths in Europe have prescribed hydrogen peroxide to over 10 million people to treat over 50 different diseases.

Hydrogen peroxide therapy works in the same manner as ozone therapy: It gives the body a high concentration of oxygen so that diseased cells die and normal cells are revitalized. Since hydrogen peroxide (H_2O_2) is simply water with one extra oxygen atom, when hydrogen peroxide is absorbed by the body, it does the same thing ozone does with its extra oxygen atom—it releases that extra atom into the blood, thereby creating a flood of oxygen.

In addition, hydrogen peroxide stimulates the movement of oxygen atoms from the bloodstream to the cells to a dramatically greater degree than is usually reached by other means. It does this by increasing oxygen and hemoglobin dissociation, thereby **maximizing the delivery of oxygen from the blood to the cells.** This delivery of the oxygen to the cells and tissues is essential for creating the oxygen boost necessary to maintaining a healthy environment that is inhospitable to disease.

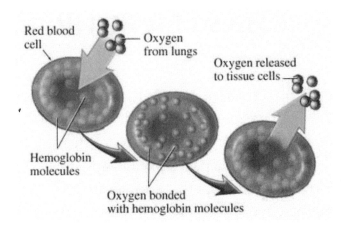

Red blood cell

Oxygen from lungs

Oxygen released to tissue cells

Hemoglobin molecules

Oxygen bonded with hemoglobin molecules

Therapeutic Use of Hydrogen Peroxide: A Brief History

During the reign of Queen Victoria over 180 years ago, when India was still a British colony, the Indian people found that hydrogen peroxide added in minute amounts to drinking water cured a variety of illnesses—from the minor ones like colds and flu all the way to serious ones like cholera and malaria. Because its use threatened the British monopoly drug sales, they hired a news reporter disguised as a doctor to *fabricate* a story about a child who supposedly died of brain damage as a result of taking hydrogen peroxide. Coming from a "doctor," the story was accepted as the truth, even if it never happened. The misinformation tactic worked and the Indian people abandoned the practice of taking hydrogen peroxide in favor of buying British drugs.

During World War I, doctors used intravenous injections of hydrogen peroxide to successfully treat pneumonia. In fact, it was a key treatment for people who became ill during the pneumonia epidemic that broke out shortly after the war.

In 1920, a British physician in India named T.H. Oliver was the first to use an intravenous infusion of hydrogen peroxide to treat a group of 25 Indian patients who were critically ill with pneumonia. Dr. Oliver's hydrogen peroxide treatment effectively cut the standard mortality rate for pneumonia from 80% to 48%.

Since then, hydrogen peroxide therapy has been studied in major medical research centers throughout the world, including Baylor University, Yale University, The University of California (Los Angeles) and Harvard University in the U.S., as well as in medical schools in Great Britain, Germany, Italy, Russia, Canada, Japan and Cuba.

Another person who is also considered a pioneer in the use of hydrogen peroxide therapy is Father Richard Willhelm. During the 1940s, he created Educational Concern for Hydrogen Peroxide (ECHO) to spread the word about the numerous benefits of hydrogen peroxide therapy. He found hydrogen peroxide especially helpful in the treatment of skin diseases, polio and mental illness brought on by bacterial infections—and believed it would prove an integral treatment for many more ailments. He created his non-profit organization hoping to inform the world about proper dosing and methods for using the treatment. However, prescription medications also became popular during the 1940s. Therefore, much of the attention that should have been placed on developing new ways to administer hydrogen peroxide became focused on the development and uses of prescription drugs instead.

In the 1950s, Dr. Reginald Holman conducted

experiments involving the use of 0.45% hydrogen peroxide concentrations added to the drinking water of rats that had cancerous tumors. The tumors completely disappeared within 15 to 60 days.

Since the late 1970s, a small group of health practitioners has advocated the use of intravenous infusions of hydrogen peroxide for a multitude of indications—including influenza, bronchitis, herpes zoster, asthmatic reactions, Epstein-Barr virus, CMV, HIV, Type II diabetes, COPD, vascular disease, arthritis, chronic pain, Alzheimer's disease, toxic dementia, Parkinson's Disease, migraine headaches, immune regulation, and even aborting an impending stroke, and destroying tumor cells. The group's rationale was based largely on the research and clinical experiences of the late Charles H. Farr, MD, PhD (1927-1998), who championed the intravenous hydrogen peroxide method, and has since been referred to as the "Father of Oxidative Medicine." In November 1986, Dr. Farr had written the landmark report titled, *"The Therapeutic Use of Intravenous Hydrogen Peroxide"*. (See the entire 11-page report at https://tinyurl. com/TherapeuticUse-IV-H2O2)

In the 1960s, European physicians began prescribing hydrogen peroxide to their patients. Before long, the use of hydrogen peroxide became an accepted part of the medical mainstream in Germany and Russia, as well as Cuba.

Although the successful treatments were widely publicized, U.S.-based physicians who tried to adopt the bio-oxidative therapies involving ozone and hydrogen peroxide were often harassed by local medical societies and threatened with the revocation of their medical licenses. As a result, hundreds of American patients flocked to foreign physicians every year seeking bio-oxidative therapies—and sadly, an untold number of Americans who had neither heard of these therapies nor had the money to travel to foreign countries to seek treatment, had to suffer needlessly or die of an untold number of diseases.

Today, despite decades of clinical success, bio-oxidative therapies are still considered "experimental" and not approved by the FDA. Over 91,000 studies attesting to the success of hydrogen peroxide therapy are presently in circulation. To see some of these studies, go to the National Institute of Health's PubMed website at www.ncbi.nlm.nih. gov/pubmed/ (enter 'hydrogen peroxide' as a search criteria).

> "If the level of hydrogen peroxide in our bodily fluids is elevated only moderately, our body becomes amazingly inhospitable to any type of pathogenic organisms."

Despite the abundance of science-backed studies supporting hydrogen peroxide therapy, a large portion of the medical community still continues to overlook—or purposely ignore—this incredibly simple and inexpensive treatment option that could potentially solve the health care crisis. To date, although over 15,000 European doctors, naturopaths and homeopaths are routinely administering medical ozone and hydrogen peroxide to millions of patients, there are fewer than 500 doctors in the U.S. who are courageous enough to use these bio-oxidative therapies in their practice. One reason for this is because information ozone and hydrogen peroxide is deliberately excluded from the curriculum in medical schools. Furthermore, medical boards do not look favorably upon licensed physicians who use bio-oxidative therapies in their medical practice, and have been known to threaten doctors with a revocation of their license—or even jail time—if they administer hydrogen peroxide or ozone.

Current Applications

Hydrogen peroxide therapy has an astounding number of applications. Alternative health practitioners, as well as researchers and doctors, have yet to find a disease that does not respond well to it—and when used properly, there are no known risks. The only people for whom hydrogen peroxide administration is not recommended are individuals who have undergone organ transplants. Hydrogen peroxide stimulates the immune system, and since the immune system attacks any foreign body that is different from what is normally present in your body, it identifies a transplanted organ as a foreign substance that needs to be eliminated. Therefore, there's a possibility that the organ could be rejected.

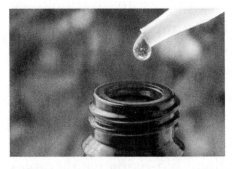

In the previous section, thirty-three major diseases were identified as having been successfully treated via ozone therapy administered through blood infusions. The following tables offer an expanded list of the diseases, bacteria, and fungi that are effectively treated by bio-oxidative therapy in general (including hydrogen peroxide).

Diseases / Ailments

AIDS	Gingivitis
Acne	Gum Disease
Allergies	Headaches
Altitude Sickness	Hepatitis
Alzheimer's Disease	Herpes
Anemia	Herpes Simplex
Angina	Herpes Zoster
Arrhythmia	HIV Infection
Arteriosclerosis	Influenza
Arthritis	Insect bites
Asthma	Leg ulcers
Bacterial Infections	Leukemia
Bronchitis	Lupus Erythematosis
Burns	Lymphoma
Cancer	Metastatic Carcinoma
Candidiasis	Migraine headaches
Cardiovascular Disease	Mononucleosis
Cerebral Vascular Disease	Multiple Sclerosis
Cholesterol (High)	Open sores and wounds
Chronic Pain	Parasitic infections
Cirrhosis of the liver	Parkinson's Disease
Cluster headaches	Periodontal Disease
Colitis	Proctitis
COPD	Prostatitis
Cystitis	Rheumatoid Arthritis
Diabetes Type II	Shingles
Diabetic Gangrene	Sinusitis
Diabetic Retinopathy	Sore Throat
Digestion Problems	Temporal Arteritis
Eczema	Trichomoniasis
Emphysema	Ulcers
Epstein-Barr infection	Vascular Diseases
Food allergies	Vascular headaches
Fungal infections	Viral infections
Fungus	Warts
Gangrene	Yeast infection

Bacteria	
Actinobacillus actinomycetermoncomitans	Legionella pneumophila
Aspergillus fumigates	Mucroraceae
Bacillus cereus	Mycobacterium leprae
Bacteroides	Neisseria gonorrhoeae
Blastomyces	Paraoccidioides
Campylobacter jejuni	Pseudomonas aeruginosa
Candida albicans	Salmonella typhi
Coccidioides	Salmonella typhimurium
Coccidioides immitis	Sporothrix
Escherichia coli	Staphylococcus aureus
Group B streptococci	Treponema pallidum
Histoplasma capsulatum	

Bio-oxidative therapy is also an effective treatment for various types of tumors as well as viruses including **Human Immunodeficiency Virus** (HIV), **Coronavirus** (SARS-CoV-2), cytomegalovirus, Lymphocytic choriomeningitis virus and Tacaribe virus.

Hydrogen Peroxide as an Alternative to Interferon

People who suffer from Multiple Sclerosis and other diseases that affect the nervous and immune systems also benefit from hydrogen peroxide therapy. Interferon drugs are often touted by medical practitioners as the best treatment option for neurological diseases, but they are expensive and are often administered through painful shots. They also come with a number of unpleasant side effects. Hydrogen peroxide therapy is an excellent option because of its ability to strengthen the immune system as a result of the boost in oxygen supply. Interestingly, the efficacy of interferon drugs comes from the fact that they, too, work by raising the body's oxygen level. Therefore, one may find that hydrogen peroxide therapy delivers many of the same benefits as interferon without the adverse side effects.

Will Hydrogen Peroxide Make Periodontal Surgery Obsolete?

People who suffer from gum disease and other mouth problems often undergo painful surgery in hopes of easing discomfort and stopping the disease from progressing. Dr. Paul Cummings once taught gum surgery techniques at the University of North Carolina, but today he relies heavily on hydrogen peroxide therapy to achieve results never before achieved. After treating about 1,000 patients with hydrogen peroxide therapy, he had a 98% success rate. Today, he is quick to report that **hydrogen peroxide therapy is more effective than periodontal surgery,** and that periodontal surgery is now rarely necessary.

One patient in particular reported that she underwent gum surgery after struggling with periodontal disease for a number of years. Her doctor performed gum surgery on a quadrant of her mouth and recommended even more surgery. Because she couldn't face the pain and expense of additional surgery, she decided to try hydrogen peroxide therapy. After using the therapy at home, she found that her gums returned to a healthy state; she no longer had pain or swelling, and her gums no longer bled or produced pus.

The possibilities of hydrogen peroxide therapy in dentistry are exciting, and many dentists have begun to recognize that it is more beneficial than surgery.

Simply brushing your teeth with a 3% hydrogen peroxide solution *(see Making a 3% Hydrogen Peroxide Solution in Chapter 5)* not only prevents gum disease but also whitens teeth and fights cavities.

"I've told many people about The One-Minute Cure book. I initially wanted to try it for periodontal problems. In two weeks, two of my deep periodontal pockets had improved (depth reduced), and none of the others were any worse. Periodontal cleaning is now done every 4 months (used to be every 3 months). Upon seeing my improvements, my hygienist wanted to know the name of the book and where to order the 35% food-grade hydrogen peroxide. She wanted this for her parents who also have periodontal problems. I would recommend it for everyone." -- Emilia B.

The Solution to Alcoholism

Another disease in which hydrogen peroxide has shown great promise is alcoholism. Alcoholism is a chronic, progressive, incurable disease involving the inability to control alcohol consumption. Alcohol creates a state of oxygen deficiency in the bodily tissues because it is a toxic agent that impairs cellular respiration. The impaired cellular respiration causes a condition called histotoxic hypoxia, which means the cells and tissues are unable to utilize or metabolize the oxygen from the bloodstream. Therefore, the cells and tissues become starved for oxygen.

Dr. P.M. Van Wulfften Palthe reported that inhalation of oxygen overcomes the effects of alcohol intoxication. Curiously enough, it was also observed that when alcoholics start taking hydrogen peroxide orally, which oxygenates the body, **they lose the craving for alcohol.** With constant use of H_2O_2, the desire for alcohol does not return. This has led some to conclude that oxygen deficiency is linked in some way to alcoholism—not just as its effect, but also the reason why the disease is often chronic and progressive. Hydrogen peroxide reverses the tissue poisoning which causes the impairment of cellular respiration in an alcoholic and restores the respiratory activity of the cells, thereby enabling them to utilize the blood oxygen again. A flood of oxygen, therefore (via hydrogen peroxide administration) arrests the disease, preventing it from progressing further.

Vodka Drinker Beats Alcoholism with H2O2 Therapy

"I purchased The One-Minute Cure book and started the regimen. I was an alcoholic at the time, and I used to drink a pint of vodka every day. The very first time I used H₂O₂, the very thought of drinking alcohol made me nauseous. I have been alcohol-free for five days now. I am sooooo happy--and I'm also saving $5.00+ a day that I used to spend on alcohol." – Anne R.

Reversing Everyday Brain Damage

Another potential benefit of using hydrogen peroxide is the reversal of the typical "slight brain damage" caused by gradual oxygen deprivation. If you live in a city where the air is oxygen-deficient—or you have an oxygen-depleting lifestyle—chances are, your brain's function has been compromised to one extent or another. Most people undergo gradual oxygen starvation without even knowing it.

Chronically unnoticed lack of oxygen causes many inexplicable illnesses such as depression, lack of energy, irritability, malaise, impaired judgment and a host of other health problems. Hydrogen peroxide administration restores an ample supply of oxygen to the brain, reverses the brain damage, and boosts energy, improves memory, alertness, concentration and even IQ.

"I Have Energy!"

"Hydrogen peroxide cured sluggishness, lack of energy and a general constant ill feeling. I started taking diluted food grade hydrogen peroxide about a month or six weeks ago and the change is amazing. I have energy! I no longer spend hours and hours and hours on the sofa. I actually do stuff. I feel so much better in general. I definitely feel as if I can breathe. " -- Jules, Palm Springs, California

The health conditions effectively treated by the proper administration of hydrogen peroxide range from serious, life-threatening diseases to minor ailments that are more bothersome than conditions that compromise health, such as acne, warts and halitosis. People even find that if they start hydrogen peroxide therapy after the onset of the flu, they feel significantly better the next day and are well by the third day. Hydrogen peroxide offers a myriad of benefits that can help you with everything from serious diseases to the common cold, and that's why it has been referred to by many as a *panacea*.

However, here's one word of caution: **Do NOT attempt to use hydrogen peroxide for disease prevention or cure until you read this entire book.** Although the FDA has given hydrogen peroxide the GRAS designation (which means *generally recognized as safe*), hydrogen peroxide is a reactive chemical that is toxic when concentrated, and can cause health hazards if not used properly. When diluted to therapeutic levels, however, it is infinitely beneficial to health. (See section titled *Home Use of Hydrogen Peroxide* on page 73 for complete instructions.)

If you choose to use hydrogen peroxide topically, it is an excellent antiseptic that can be used to clean cuts and other wounds. You can apply the **pharmaceutical grade** 3% hydrogen peroxide—the kind that is available at your local drugstore (for external use only)—directly onto the skin. Many people find it especially effective in the treatment of acne and persistent wounds due to diabetes. If you plan to use hydrogen peroxide internally, you will need to use a food-grade formula, about which you will learn more in the next chapter. Finally, you may choose to administer **food-grade** hydrogen peroxide mist as a nasal spray or **(see instructions for using this method on page 87)** through the use of a vaporizer or nebulizer to combat breathing and sinus-related problems—and stop COVID-19 dead in its tracks.

What Doctors are Saying

While the medical community as a whole does not yet accept the validity of ozone and hydrogen peroxide therapy—at least not openly— there is a growing number of physicians and researchers in the U.S. who promote its use. Many proclaim the benefits of hydrogen peroxide therapy as nothing less than *the greatest healing miracle of all time.*

In a 4200-word article by Dr. David G. Williams, one of the world's leading authorities on natural healing, he praised the health benefits of hydrogen peroxide, stating, "I'll admit I was skeptical when I first learned about using H_2O_2 orally or intravenously. This healthy dose of skepticism, however, led to a great deal of investigation, clinical work and experimentation. And while I realize a large majority of readers will probably never be convinced that H_2O_2 is a safe and effective compound, I am. **Hydrogen peroxide is safe, readily available and dirt cheap. And best of all, it works!**"

Dr. William Campbell Douglass, a fourth generation physician and proponent of the therapeutic use of H_2O_2, wrote that hydrogen "peroxide is certainly a universal agent which can almost always be tried for an illness, often with great success."

In an article for a publication called *Alternatives*, Dr. Kurt Donsbach wrote: "One ounce of 35% hydrogen peroxide (per gallon of water) in a vaporizer every night in an emphysemic's bedroom, and they will breathe freer than they have breathed in years! I do this for my lung cancer patients." Dr. Donsbach also uses hydrogen peroxide in every one of his cancer patients.

In Mexico, health practitioners at the Gerson Institute and La Gloria Clinic enthusiastically recommend hydrogen peroxide therapy to their patients because they tried it at their respective centers and found numerous benefits.

Throughout the rest of the world, hundreds of doctors attest to the benefits of hydrogen peroxide therapy. Dr. Charles H. Farr—referred to as the "Father of Oxidative Medicine"—recognizes it as an effective way to rid patients of diseases once thought incurable.

People Saved from the Brink of Death by Hydrogen Peroxide

This is an excerpt from a real-life case study. Names have been changed for privacy reasons.

Dr. Lance Moriarty, the Director of a medical clinic in Nairobi, Kenya (where 1 out of every 8 people is infected with AIDS or HIV), reported that "Patients have literally been dragged back from the brink of death" from the use of hydrogen peroxide. When administered to 50 patients who were suffering from AIDS or the HIV virus, 30 of them went into immediate remission—and the rest of the patients reported an increase in stamina and a sense of well-being they never had before. This success rate is unheard of in the medical and pharmaceutical world where AIDS is still considered incurable! Dr. Moriarty went on to say that whenever the one-minute cure is administered throughout the community, "People come back to life! It blows my mind!"

One of the most notable physicians to recommend the use of hydrogen peroxide therapy is the late Dr. Christiaan Barnard. In 1986, Dr. Barnard, who is most well-known for completing the first successful heart transplant surgery, began recommending hydrogen peroxide therapy to his patients. He had been using it himself to treat arthritis and other ailments related to aging—and was impressed by its effectiveness. Dr. Barnard was ridiculed so heavily by members of the medical community that he ceased claiming any affiliation with the hundreds of doctors who recommended the therapy. However, he did not retract the fact that he was using hydrogen peroxide therapy himself. Though oxygen therapy is still not considered legitimate by the medical community at large, numerous other health practitioners use it to cure virtually all diseases—from cancer to diabetes to heart disease.

"She should already be dead ..."
if it weren't for hydrogen peroxide

This is an excerpt from a real-life case study. Names have been changed for privacy reasons.

Carla Trueman had the worst possible case of lupus, with severe complications—including inflammation and swelling of the brain, open sores and nephritis, which almost led to kidney failure. Since she was part of a medical study being conducted at a university, the university specialist prescribed a drug called Cytoxan for treatment, but because of the many possible side effects of the drug, she refused to take it. Instead, she began self-administering hydrogen peroxide every day. Her case was later presented at the medical school, and when they examined her and found no sign of lupus, they questioned whether she ever had lupus at all.

~ CHAPTER FIVE ~

In a previous chapter, ozone therapy was described as being powerful in curing even the deadliest diseases, particularly AIDS. It's worthwhile noting that most of the benefits attributed to the administration of medical ozone can also be attributed to the administration of hydrogen peroxide as well, since **ozone is transformed into hydrogen peroxide in the body.** The mechanism by which hostile microorganisms are eradicated by hydrogen peroxide is the same as with ozone blood infusion. Like ozone, hydrogen peroxide kills viruses and other pathogens by oxidation as it spreads through the tissues of the human body. At the same time, the oxygen boost revitalizes normal cells.

Hydrogen peroxide is safe if used correctly—and best of all, its health benefits are accompanied by practically no known risks.

Home Use of Hydrogen Peroxide

Before you decide on how you plan to self-administer hydrogen peroxide therapy, it is critical that you understand the different grades of hydrogen peroxide available. The grades are as follows:

- **3% Pharmaceutical Grade:** This is the hydrogen peroxide that's available at your local drugstore. It is for external use only and should not be ingested because it contains a number of stabilizers including acetanilide, phenol, sodium stagnate, and tetrasodium phosphate.

- **6% Beautician Grade:** This hydrogen peroxide grade is used by hair stylists to bleach hair. It is not to be ingested because it contains stabilizers as well as bleach.

- **30% Reagent grade:** This has uses in a number of scientific experiments, but it contains stabilizers and is not for internal use.

- **30–32% Electronic Grade:** This hydrogen peroxide is used to clean electronics and is not for internal use.

- **35% Technical Grade:** This hydrogen peroxide is similar to Reagent grade—but it is more concentrated and contains phosphorus to neutralize chlorine in the water that is added to dilute it.

- **35% Food-Grade: This is the only grade of hydrogen peroxide recommended for internal use.** It's commonly used in the production of dairy products like milk and eggs. It is also sprayed onto the foil lining of products like juice and acts as an antiseptic. You can purchase this formula in pints, quarts, gallons, and drums. (See Resources section for stores and online retailers that carry 35% food-grade hydrogen peroxide.)

  IMPORTANT NOTE: The 35% strength must be diluted before being taken internally. (See instructions below)

- **90%:** This hydrogen peroxide is used as a source of oxygen in rocket fuel.

Internal Use of Hydrogen Peroxide

If you plan to ingest hydrogen peroxide as part of your therapy, clearly, you will want to **use only the 35% food-grade formula.** At this strength, however, the product must be handled with care as it will oxidize skin tissue immediately on contact, and you will sense this as a burning sensation. Should it come in direct contact with your skin, flush it out with water immediately. **Under no circumstances should you ingest undiluted hydrogen peroxide.** Even at slightly over 10% strength, *undiluted* hydrogen peroxide can potentially cause neurological damage. Be careful to dilute hydrogen peroxide properly using the suggested protocol in the table below.

Many people find that the most convenient way to dispense hydrogen peroxide is with a glass bottle via eyedropper cap. Once you fill the glass bottle, label it "35% Food Grade Hydrogen Peroxide" in order to prevent accidental undiluted use), store the remaining hydrogen peroxide in the freezer, out of the reach of children. If you don't use all the hydrogen peroxide that is contained in the bottle with eyedropper cap, you can leave it in the refrigerator until you administer your next dose.

Day	Number of Drops of 35% Food-Grade H$_2$O$_2$ Diluted in 6-8 Ounces Distilled Water	Times Administered Daily
1	3	3
2	4	3
3	5	3
4	6	3
5	7	3
6	8	3
7	9	3
8	10	3
9	11	3
10	12	3
11	13	3
12	14	3
13	15	3
14	16	3
15	17	3
16	18	3
17	19	3
18	20	3
19	21	3
20	22	3
21	23	3
22	24	3
23	25	3

The table on the previous page provides a suggested schedule for your hydrogen peroxide therapy. Each dose takes less than 1 minute to administer. Use only distilled water to dilute hydrogen peroxide; do not use water that has been chlorinated. The drops should be diluted in 6 to 8 ounces of water.

Tap or mineral water contains dissolved minerals that will react with the extra oxygen; hence, diluting the food-grade hydrogen peroxide in distilled water is recommended.

In addition, Vitamin C, iron and fats in the stomach change hydrogen peroxide into super-oxide free radicals, which can damage the lining of your stomach. Hence, it's important to take the diluted food-grade hydrogen peroxide on an empty stomach—*one hour before* a meal or *3 hours after* a meal.

When you have completed the 23-day regimen in the table, gradually decrease the dosage by one drop a day until you get to the *maintenance* dose of 3 drops (diluted in 6-8 ozs of distilled water) 3 times a day. This suggested protocol is based on years of experience and success stories from thousands of users.

Food-grade hydrogen peroxide is very inexpensive (approximately $13 for a 16 oz. bottle). Therefore, the maintenance dose of 3 drops in water 3 times a day will cost only 1½ cents per day, and the maximum dose of 25 drops in water 3 times a day will cost only 12 cents per day.

If you have a serious condition, you may wish to try taking 25 drops three times daily for one to three weeks during the beginning portion of the maintenance phase before tapering down to 25 drops two times per day for up to six months. Otherwise, you can reduce the maintenance schedule to between 5 and 15 drops based on how you are feeling.

Hydrogen peroxide is not tasteless, so once you start adding more and more drops to your distilled water, you may discover that it tastes like bleach. Some people find it impossible to drink water containing 25 drops because of the unpleasant taste. Others find that chewing sugar-free gum (with no artificial flavors or sweeteners) after drinking the solution solves the problem.

If you find the taste unpleasant, try diluting the hydrogen peroxide with six to eight ounces of milk, aloe vera, or watermelon juice instead of water. If you are still bothered by a bleachy aftertaste, cut down on the number of drops you put into each glass and increase the number of glasses you drink each day. Or simply go up to the number of drops you can tolerate—and supplement that oral H_2O_2 regimen by also drinking *ozonated water* (see page 52) or *inhaling nebulized hydrogen peroxide* (see page 89), both of which can also super-oxygenate the body and accelerate healing.

As previously mentioned, it is important that you **take the diluted food-grade hydrogen peroxide on an empty stomach.** The best times are at least one hour before mealtime and/or at least three hours after mealtime. Hydrogen peroxide will react with food's bacteria in your stomach, and the result is excess foaming, nausea and possibly vomiting.

Although it is not common, you may experience symptoms including nausea, fatigue, diarrhea and cold or flu-like symptoms as your body attempts to expel large amounts of dead cells. This phase is what is referred to as the *healing crisis*, which is the body's reaction to the removal of disease-causing or toxic conditions. It doesn't happen in the majority of cases, but some may experience it, as well as a range of other minor symptoms. Do not stop your regimen if you experience these symptoms; you may be uncomfortable for a day or two, but it means the therapy is working.

Although uncommon, you may find that your skin may break out for a few days or longer, or you may even develop boils or other types of skin inflammations. These symptoms mean that your body is working hard to get rid of toxins, and they will pass within a few days. Also, if you have certain viruses or bacteria in your stomach, like streptococcus, you might feel nauseous for the first few days of therapy. It is very important that you continue your hydrogen peroxide therapy; do not discontinue use if you experience bothersome symptoms. Keep in mind that your body is ridding itself of disease and toxins, and you will begin to feel much better within a few days.

On April 8, 2009, 41-year-old single mom, Randie (from Canada), started undergoing a "healing crisis" which she reported to us after starting the H_2O_2 regimen. Her skin started oozing a yellow liquid, which hardened into a mask. Seven days later, after the healing crisis had passed, we received an ecstatic e-mail from Randie, accompanied by 5 pictures of herself – before, during and after taking the H_2O_2. An excerpt of her e-mail follows:

"The best part is I am back! My skin looks so wonderful! I have never looked so smooth and clear since I was 10 years old! All my acne scars are gone and so are my wrinkles! I love it, love it, love it! The best part also is this: I started this whole process because since the age of 17, I have suffered from IBS (irritable bowel syndrome) but I have had no problems since the 4th day of my H_2O_2 drops. I used to be on the toilet 7-9 times a day with the runs, now I have a good solid stool in the mornings and that is that. I am thrilled!

"To top off all this good news is something even more amazing. I can **smell**. I lost my sense of smell when I was 6 years old after a bad case of pneumonia. I am now 41 years old—and smelling food for what seems like the first time ever! Food really does taste like it smells, something I have missed out on for over 30 years. I love the smell of popcorn and garlic!!! I can't wait to smell flowers in the spring."

"Thank you so very much for printing this book. You have changed my life forever. By the way, I am not the only one going through changes. I also put my 3 children on the H2o2 drops. Rashes have cleared, acne is a thing of the past, better sleep and more positive attitude from my teenagers— all make a world of difference. We are all just happier."

If you want your drinking water to taste like fresh spring water, put seven drops of 35% food-grade hydrogen peroxide into a gallon of water, and shake the bottle. You can keep this mixture in the refrigerator and drink it as much as you would like.

Intravenous Injection of Hydrogen Peroxide

Oral ingestion of diluted hydrogen peroxide is not the only way H_2O_2 can be administered for therapeutic purposes. It can also be administered by a trained physician via intravenous injection. Much of the research and scientific literature extolling the benefits of hydrogen peroxide was derived from studies involving intravenous injection. This form of bio-oxidative therapy has been used for the last several decades, and was found to be effective in treating pneumonia as far back as post-World War I days.

Intravenous injections of hydrogen peroxide are regarded as being particularly convenient for health practitioners to recommend because they can be used in conjunction with almost any type of therapy used to treat diseases, although they do need to be administered separately from other treatments.

Intravenous injections of hydrogen peroxide work just like oral administration of H_2O_2—that is, their mechanism of action is based on giving tissues a healthy boost of oxygen. With intravenous injections, however, the oxygen is delivered directly into the bloodstream and also causes the body to produce oxygen in response to the hydrogen peroxide. It is, therefore, a viable treatment option on its own.

Intravenous injections of hydrogen peroxide have proven particularly useful in treating emphysema. Emphysema is most often caused by smoking, and it attacks the alveoli, the small air sacks within the lungs. Currently, there is no widely-recognized cure for the disease, and patients have only been able to find some relief from their symptoms through conventional medical techniques. Emphysema causes one's heart to work too hard to circulate blood, and death often ensues because of eventual heart failure. Although breathing difficulties of emphysema patients have been effectively relieved by running a vaporizer (containing one ounce of food-grade hydrogen peroxide in a gallon of water) throughout the night, eliminating all the other drastic effects of emphysema has been a challenging task. In this regard, intravenous injection of hydrogen peroxide has become the choice therapy, yielding the most amazing results.

When injected, the hydrogen peroxide goes to the diseased areas of the lungs and begins to bubble between the layer of mucus and the lining of the lungs. The patient coughs up the mucus as the doctor regulates the amount of hydrogen peroxide that is administered intravenously. Many patients have reported that intravenous injections have improved their breathing so much that they no longer need oxygen tanks and wheelchairs.

To find a physician trained to administer intravenous injections of hydrogen peroxide, refer to the Hydrogen Peroxide Therapy Practitioner Directory in the Resources section of this book (page 143).

Unheard-Of Remarkable Recovery from Emphysema

This is a real-life case study. The names of both the doctor and the patient have been changed for privacy reasons.

Rick Dorrington was brought to Dr. Michael Erwin's clinic with a terminal case of emphysema. He was extremely thin, wheelchair-bound, and had a portable oxygen tank with him at all times because he had so much trouble breathing. Dr. Erwin began administering hydrogen peroxide intravenously. After only 4 treatments, Rick no longer had to use his wheelchair, and he discarded the oxygen tank altogether. He was also able to sleep flat on his bed without having to be propped up because of breathing difficulties -- and his appetite returned, accompanied by a healthy weight gain. This remarkable recovery is unheard of among emphysema patients!

Making a 3% Hydrogen Peroxide Solution

There are times when it would be convenient for you to keep a 3% strength food-grade hydrogen peroxide on hand because at this strength, it has many uses that produce countless benefits—in addition to the benefits that are derived from the dosing regimen described earlier. This should not be confused with the 3% hydrogen peroxide that you can find at your local drugstore because that pharmaceutical grade is for *external use* only and should not be ingested.

In order to make a 3% solution that can be ingested, you must start with 35% food-grade hydrogen peroxide and dilute it according to the way it will be used. Whenever I handle a bottle of 35% food-grade hydrogen peroxide, I always wear rubber gloves while handling the bottle and associated equipment. That's because, as mentioned previously, the 35% concentration, if spilled, will oxidize skin tissue on contact, cause a burning sensation—and it will most likely turn your skin white temporarily (but will return to normal in a day or two). To start, pour one ounce of 35% food-grade hydrogen peroxide into a pint jar, and add 11 ounces of distilled water (ratio: 1 part 35% food-grade hydrogen peroxide to 11 parts distilled water). This will yield 12 ounces of 3% hydrogen peroxide. Make sure you label it "3% Food Grade Hydrogen Peroxide" to distinguish it from the 35% strength.

If you prefer to skip the task of diluting your 35% food-grade hydrogen peroxide down to 3%, you can just purchase the commercially available 3% food-grade hydrogen peroxide, which costs only about $8.00 for a 16-oz bottle.

You can use the diluted (or store-bought) 3% solution in a variety of ways, and you may find it convenient to store the unused portion in the refrigerator. If you wish to ingest the 3% food-grade hydrogen peroxide, you will need to dilute the solution further. However, absorbing 3% food-grade hydrogen peroxide through the mucous membranes, the lungs, and the skin produces many remarkable health benefits. The list below, although far from being exhaustive, provides some of the external uses of 3% hydrogen peroxide.

The Gums and Teeth

A 3% hydrogen peroxide solution can be used at full strength as a mouthwash, or it can be mixed with baking soda for use as toothpaste to fight cavities and gum disease, in addition to whitening teeth. In fact, the popular teeth whitening products on the market are effective because of their hydrogen peroxide content. The advanced action employed by the expensive ampoule-based teeth whitening systems can be duplicated at home by dipping cotton swabs into the 3% hydrogen peroxide solution and using them to gently target specific teeth. This safely whitens natural teeth optimally and safely lifts stains from porcelain crowns and veneers. You can do this twice a day, preferably after brushing your teeth. Do not rinse the hydrogen peroxide out after applying it with the cotton swabs, and do not drink or eat for 20 minutes after application so as not to hinder the optimal contact time.

Three tablespoons of a 3% hydrogen peroxide solution and a quart of chlorine-free (preferably distilled) water can be used as an enema or douche, which will ward off "bad" bacteria. It will kill anaerobic bacteria in the rectum and colon and bacterial infections and yeast in the vagina. Hydrogen peroxide can also be used at 3% strength or diluted with warm water as a foot soak for athlete's foot and diabetes-related ailments.

Absorbing Hydrogen Peroxide Through the Skin

A particularly simple way to absorb hydrogen peroxide through your skin is to bathe in it. Try adding 1 to 8 pints of the 3% solution to a bathtub full of warm water. The water will cause your pores to open, allowing your body to absorb some of the hydrogen peroxide. You may not wish to try this method close to bedtime, however, because the boost of oxygen may energize and keep you awake. Some people have used hydrogen peroxide baths to rid themselves of boils, fungus or other skin infections. (Other people have also used a pint of 35% food-grade hydrogen peroxide in a tub of water, instead of 1 to 8 pints of the 3% solution, and have reported a host of other benefits including prematurely gray hair returning to its original color.)

A foot bath using full strength 3% hydrogen peroxide has been used as an effective treatment for athlete's foot. Diabetics have been relieved of circulation problems by soaking their feet for half an hour in a foot bath consisting of 1 pint of 3% hydrogen peroxide and a gallon of warm water.

Another topical use of 3% hydrogen peroxide—in addition to its common use as an antiseptic for cuts and wounds—is as a remedy for acne and a variety of other skin conditions. Applying 3% hydrogen peroxide full strength to the affected areas once or twice a day with a cotton ball or swab has shown surprisingly rapid results.

Gray Hair Returning to Its Original Color

"I am a Certified Hypnotherapist and Herbalist. I am sixty-five years old. We need brave people like you to lead us to the ultimate freedom of human soul. After 3 weeks of using the H202, a lot people, when they walk in to my store, say my gray hair is changing back to my natural color black. They want to know what am I using. I think this is the 'Panacea' we all are waiting for—the cure or prevention for all diseases. I'm ordering 25 copies of the book so that whenever people notice my hair changing color, and me looking younger, I will tell them to read the book! — S. Ghazi, Los Angeles, California

Inhalation Method

One popular and convenient method for absorbing 3% hydrogen peroxide solution is through a nasal spray pump or spray bottle. You can purchase a nasal spray bottle at a medical supply or beauty supply store. As an alternative, you can buy a product contained in a nasal spray at your local drugstore, empty the bottle's contents, wash it thoroughly with soap and water, and fill it with the 3% hydrogen peroxide solution. Pump the 3% contents of the spray bottle/nasal spray—5 to 10 pumps into your mouth while inhaling the mist deeply into your lungs. Repeat this twice in the morning and twice at night. If you have been feeling sick, administer the procedure every four to six hours. If you have a virus, use the spray every two hours. Usually, the virus will be gone within 36 to 48 hours, depending on its severity. If you have had a virus for a while, you may find that it takes a week or longer for the treatment to take effect.

Although the amount of hydrogen peroxide administered via the spray bottle/nasal spray pump method is minute, it is very effective in alleviating numerous conditions. Countless people have claimed that this method has drastically improved their quality of life by getting rid of ailments ranging from colds to melanoma to stiff muscles. One person reported having cured prostate cancer in a month, and another reported that a happy side-effect of using hydrogen peroxide nasal spray is improved self esteem. This is not hard to believe since a boost of oxygen often makes people feel energized. Some even find that they must use it during the day because spraying close to bedtime makes them too awake and alert to go to sleep.

Word-Renowned Beverly Hills Cosmetic Surgeon Prefers the Inhalation Method

Dr. Simon O., a Beverly Hills cosmetic surgeon to celebrities, is a strong believer in food-grade hydrogen peroxide therapy. His preferred mode of administration is the inhalation method because he said, "The hydrogen peroxide goes straight to your lungs, where it can benefit your health immediately."

An effective way to administer hydrogen peroxide to the lungs is to add it to a vaporizer or humidifier. Many people find that adding 12 ounces of 3% hydrogen peroxide to one gallon of water in a vaporizer that is run all night, drastically improves their breathing and wards off colds and the flu. Some people even note that they no longer snore.

Dr. Kurt Donsbach, D.C., N.D., Ph.D., the visionary inventor, healer—and founder of the 3 largest wholistic hospitals in the world, specializing in cancer and degenerative diseases—administers this exact protocol to his patients with emphysema and lung cancer. In his own words: "I will give you, in 30 seconds, a 20% benefit to all emphysemics. Twelve ounces of 3% food grade hydrogen peroxide (per gallon of water) in a vaporizer every night in an emphysemic's bedroom, and they will breathe freer than they have breathed in years! I do this for my lung cancer patients. Patients who could not lie down in bed to sleep can lie down after one night of breathing the vapors of hydrogen peroxide. It's amazing. It's a very simple thing to do."

Terminal Lung Cancer Healed through Food-Grade H₂O₂ in Humidifier

"I've reported in this blog before that my mother beat lung cancer. Gone completely. She was given six months to live. My brother, who took care of her, said that the only thing she did religiously was take hydrogen peroxide. Essentially, it is water with an extra molecule of oxygen. Studies conclusively prove that oxygen shrinks cancer.

"My mother started with this book: The One-Minute Cure: The Secret to Healing Virtually All Diseases and it explains that use of "food grade hydrogen peroxide" fills the entire body with extra oxygen and makes the "entire environment" so healthy that it has the ability to heal itself of ALL Disease. My mother was given six months to live, but a year and half later, the cancer was gone completely from her lungs! It turns out she was putting the food-grade hydrogen peroxide into a vaporizer, as explained in the book) and breathing it in all night. And of all the things she tried, this was the one thing she did every single day no matter what." — C. Holmes, Los Angeles, California

Nebulized Hydrogen Peroxide

When the first edition of this book was published in 2008, it didn't include mention of the inhalation method involving nebulized hydrogen peroxide. Now, since COVID-19 has dominated the global health landscape, it has become imperative to include its discussion in this second edition.

In order to appreciate the significance of nebulized hydrogen peroxide, here's a brief background:

Nebulized hydrogen peroxide as a therapy for eradicating viruses was originally conceptualized by Charles Farr MD—"The Father of Oxidative Medicine"—in the early 1990s.

It was subsequently researched and prescribed by Frank Shallenberger MD for resolving respiratory viruses, acute viral infections, flu viruses and—beginning in 2020—the coronavirus.

Dr. David Brownstein has used this safe, inexpensive nebulized hydrogen peroxide therapy for 25 years with no adverse effects. As of the time of this writing, he has successfully treated over 207 COVID-19 patients with nebulized hydrogen peroxide, and published a case paper about this treatment in the July 2020 issue of *Science, Public Health Policy and The Law.*

What is nebulized hydrogen peroxide? It's a diluted concentration of food-grade hydrogen peroxide placed in a nebulizer, a device that is able to convert a liquid into tiny, microscopic bubbles. These extremely small bubbles—which resemble smoke escaping from the nebulizer—can be inhaled into the deepest regions of the lungs without any discomfort or irritation.

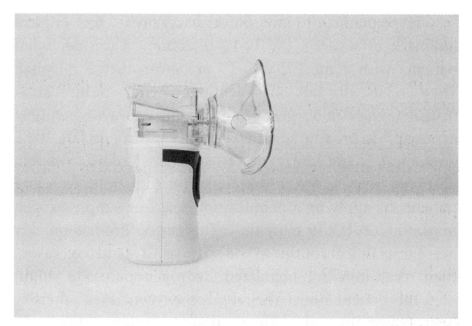

Nebulizers have long been utilized for asthmatics to get medication to open their lungs. Dr. Shallenberger further noticed that nebulizers have a systemic effect, which delivers the medication—in this case, the food-grade hydrogen peroxide—throughout the body far beyond the lungs.

What is nebulized hydrogen peroxide's mechanism of action? It appears that the peroxide forms a powerful signaling function that stimulates the immune system to defeat whatever viral threat it encounters. Your immune cells actually produce hydrogen peroxide on their own, which explains how they kill cells that have been infected with a virus. When one's immune cells are overwhelmed—such as the case with COVID-19—nebulized hydrogen peroxide merely boosts the hydrogen peroxide level in your immune cells, thereby enabling them to perform their natural function more effectively.

Hypoxemia--or low blood oxygen--is the clinical hallmark of severe COVID-19 infection. Consider what patients with acute COVID-19 are given in the hospital: They are usually put on a ventilator, which pumps air—usually with extra oxygen—into patients' airways when they are unable to breathe adequately on their own. In late 2020, doctors at Skåne University Hospital in Malmö, Sweden, observed that oxygenation could be improved in some patients by applying a nebulization mask or simple oxygen mask to COVID-19 patients. This procedure has quickly become a clinical routine at the hospital. It stands to reason, then, that inhaling nebulized hydrogen peroxide might help the patient boost their body's oxygen levels, thereby neutralizing any and all viruses that are present in the body.

Among the treatment options that have demonstrated high levels of effectiveness and success with COVID-19—including hydroxychloroquine, the MATH+ and I-MASK+ protocols, Ivermectin, quercetin and zinc—"the single most effective intervention for those who have acute COVID-19" is nebulized hydrogen peroxide, according to Dr. Joseph Mercola. Nebulized hydrogen peroxide is Dr. Mercola's favorite intervention for acute viral illnesses in general, because he strongly believes it would "prevent the majority of people from dying from COVID-19 if used."

It might be worth noting that Dr. Mercola has been discredited and maligned by government authorities, the medical establishment and mainstream media, who call him a "super-spreader of COVID-19 misinformation". With regards to Dr. Mercola's claims regarding nebulized hydrogen peroxide as a home remedy for COVID-19, one media source said, "According to the Federal Trade Commission (FTC), there is no study known to exist that supports that."

So the question remains: Does nebulized hydrogen peroxide prevent and/or cure COVID-19?

Government authorities, regulatory agencies—and even social media—prohibit anyone from making this claim. Such entities routinely censor, ban or shut down any articles, videos, and content that make claims of preventing or curing COVID-19. Case in point: Dr. Joseph Mercola was forced to remove all references to COVID-19 from his website, as well as remove the entire archive of health articles that had taken him 25 years to create.

Therefore, it's up to you to understand what hydrogen peroxide does in the body—as explained in the preceding chapters of this book—and decide for yourself if the science and evidence validates the use of nebulized hydrogen peroxide therapy for preventing and curing COVID-19. As stated in Chapter 3, it is not uncommon for the pharmaceutical industry to disseminate negative propaganda and sometimes even fabricate reports of adverse events or death from the use of H_2O_2 therapy—all in the name of protecting its financial interests.

Dr. Farr's original therapy for eradicating viruses primarily involved an intravenous administration of hydrogen peroxide, which is beyond the logistical (and perhaps financial) capacity of most people. This may be one reason why that original hydrogen peroxide therapy has not gained much traction. Years later, the nebulized hydrogen peroxide method developed by Dr. Frank Shallenberger was found to be almost as effective as intravenous H_2O_2 in eradicating viruses, can be performed at home, and is affordable and accessible to most people.

Nebulized hydrogen peroxide can be highly effective, and it also has no known side effects, when used properly. Dr. Thomas Levy, who's an advocate of Dr. Frank Shallenberger's protocol, uses full-strength hydrogen peroxide when using a nebulizer. Dr. Mercola, on the other hand, recommends diluting the 3% food-grade hydrogen peroxide (0.1 percent, which is 30 times less concentrated than regular drugstore 3% H_2O_2)—and adding a pinch of Himalayan salt to add electrolytes and protect the lungs from potential damage.

How to Use Nebulized Hydrogen Peroxide

Nebulized hydrogen peroxide is extremely easy to administer. Simply put a small quantity of 3% food-grade hydrogen peroxide in the nebulization chamber of the nebulizer, press the ON button, and begin inhaling the fine mist of H_2O_2 "bubbles" (using the plastic 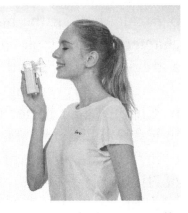 face mask that comes with the nebulizer). Inhale normally as though you're just breathing pure air. For preventive purposes, inhale for 3-5 minutes a day. For early onset or treatment of a virus or an acute viral infection, inhale for 10–15 minute sessions, 4 times a day, until symptomatic relief is realized.

As it is a completely non-toxic therapy, nebulized

hydrogen peroxide can be administered as often as desired for preventive purposes.

Note: For most adults, the 3% food-grade concentration can be used full-strength in the nebulization chamber, without diluting. This optimizes the degree and rapidity of anti-viral and anti-pathogen effect, according to Dr. Levy. However, if you wish to dilute the 3% H_2O_2 to a 0.1% concentration, as recommended by Dr. Mercola, you can dilute 1/4 teaspoon 3% H_2O_2 to 7-1/2 teaspoons filtered water, and add a pinch of Himalayan salt for electrolytes.

Portable nebulizers are fairly inexpensive (approximately $40). BestPortableNebulizer.com sells a high-quality portable nebulizer at half the price of similar models sold at Amazon and other retailers.

A Word About Anaerobic and Aerobic Bacteria

You may be concerned about using hydrogen peroxide as an enema or douche because both the colon and vagina hold a number of necessary or "good" bacteria that might be destroyed by oxygenation. You might also be wondering if ingesting hydrogen peroxide will also remove the necessary bacteria that live in your stomach to aid in digestion. Hydrogen peroxide does not harm your body's necessary bacteria because "good" bacteria are aerobic, which means they flourish in oxygen-rich environments. Disease-causing bacteria are most often anaerobic, which means they fare much better in environments with less oxygen.

Cancer of Pharynx — One Month to Live — Healed!

A French Canadian man named Yves C. bought *The One-Minute Cure* eBook for his wife who had cancer of the pharynx. On July 11, 2009, he sent the following e-mail:

"Hello, I bought your *One-Minute Cure* ebook, used it for my wife who has since been cured from a cancer of the pharynx. Last March, she was told by doctors that her cancer was not operable and incurable and that she has only one month to live. It is now 3 and half months since the bad news and she is at home recovering well. Thank you—the one-minute cure works!"

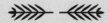

Thyroid Cancer Cured! And COVID? Not today!

Earl B. reported that he got cured of thyroid cancer using the hydrogen peroxide therapy (maintenance dose). His stunning results convinced him to purchase dozens of copies of *The One-Minute Cure* book to give away to everyone he knew who was suffering from cancer. In addition, when the coronavirus pandemic happened, all members of his immediate family got COVID-19 in the fall of 2020 -- except him, and he attributes that to the H_2O_2 that keeps his immune system strong.

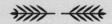

Wife's Late-Stage Breast Cancer Healed
— Friend's Emphysema Gone, Too!

In 2008, Ross Edwards's wife, Diane, was diagnosed with late-stage breast cancer. The tumor inside her was growing rapidly, and her doctor was trying to get her to have chemo—but but both Ross and Diane didn't want it for her because they knew chemo kills not just cancer cells but also the healthy cells. On November 11, 2008, Ross came across the Cancer Cure Video online, and after watching it, he had great hope again -- and ordered *The One-Minute Cure* book. He then searched for the food-grade hydrogen peroxide that the book talked about—but he couldn't fine it in Australia. Companies in the US are prohibited by aviation laws from shipping it by air -- they can only ship by land or boat. He begged us to send him the H_2O_2 from the States as quickly as possible and he promised to cover all costs since he and his wife were desperate. On November 28, we found a source of food-grade hydrogen peroxide in the Queensland Area -- a man named Robert, who ran a small clinic in Brisbane and manufactured the food-grade H_2O_2. When Ross called him, Robert not only agreed to supply him with the H_2O_2, but also offered to come to Ross's house, meet his wife, Diane, and help her administer the H_2O_2 for her cancer.

By December 28, as a result of the H_2O_2 therapy, there was a 25% reduction in the size of Diane's tumor. Ross declared that the food-grade H_2O_2 was "the best stuff in the world" and he began telling everyone he knew about *The One-Minute Cure.* By January 20, 2009, he had 7 of his friends taking it, too, for various ailments.

Six weeks after Diane started the H₂O₂ therapy, she was declared cancer-free! Ross also reported that his neighbor, who had emphysema, had no energy and was pretty much a shut-in imprisoned by her oxygen tank. A few weeks after taking H₂O₂, she got rid of her oxygen tank and was ready to go bowling!

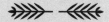

No Trace of Cancer Found

Linda F. had a cancerous tumor surgically removed. But she had reservations because: "The doctors weren't sure if all the cancer cells were taken out." She read *The One-Minute Cure* book, and began using the hydrogen peroxide therapy when she came home from the hospital. She drank the diluted H₂O₂ faithfully, and she noticed that the arthritis in her lower back was suddenly gone, the arthritis in both kneecaps were gone, hand circulation went back to "normal warmth" (not cold like before), her varicose veins were fading gradually, and the neuropathic pain in both feet was slowly going away. On her last MRI (September 14), **not a trace of cancer was found.** The doctors were surprised, but she wasn't because she knew if there were any cancer cells left, they'd be gone -- thanks to the H₂O₂.

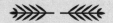

Stage 3 Leukemia Reversed

I ordered The *One-Minute Cure book* to find out if this is bogus information. I was a level 3 leukemia patient when I started using the info in this book, and one month later, I am at level 0. I only did one-third of what this book suggests and had fantastic results. If you have cancer or any disease, please do yourself a favor and read this book." — Frieda L., Amazon Verified Purchaser of *The One-Minute Cure* book

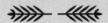

Throat Cancer - Doctors Baffled
Uncle Should Have Died a Long Time Ago!

"I just called my uncle (who has throat cancer) to tell him about hydrogen peroxide and I got all excited about it. I had read here that it had cured some people's cancers, etc., and he just laughed, then said, 'Tara, that's why my cancer is in remission!' He said he had stumbled upon this treatment accidentally, when twenty years ago he swallowed some hydrogen peroxide (not on purpose) while brushing his teeth one day. Then he said, 'It just made me feel better, so I continued to do it.' Since then, he's been drinking one 16 ounce glass of water with a little hydrogen peroxide every day ... The doctors are 'baffled', because they think he should have died a long time ago. After reading about this therapy, then talking to my uncle, a lot more lives could be saved if we dropped the propaganda and started having open discussions about human health, irrelevant of money and power." — Tara, Los Angeles, California

Advanced Stage IV Lymphoma - Cancerous Tumor Disappeared

"My husband has been battling a rare Lymphoma since 2012. He started at an advanced stage IV, on both sides of the diaphragm, including in the colon. There was no known treatment for this type, so he went into a clinical trial at MD Anderson. He was pulled after 6 months due to cardiac complications and was found clean when he was re staged —with the exception of a large active lymph node in his right groin. He has since had 3 different chemo protocols trying to eradicate this very resistant tumor. Nothing has worked ..UNTIL.... I was praying out loud in the car on my way to work in March of 18, asking God if there was anything I could do to eradicate this cancer, please direct me to it and give me the ability to understand and skills implement it. I got into my office, turned on my computer, and in the right lower corner a box popped up that said "A Cure for Cancer"... Then, I found *The One-Minute Cure* book, started implementing it for my husband and in June 2018...the very resistant cancerous tumor in his groin was now *undetectable!* God's blessing and evidence based that The One Minute Cure WORKS!!! My husband is living proof! I give God the praise for directing me to it. I have bought over 15 books and have given them to various people that are fighting different illnesses. IT WORKS!!!!" -- Ludie, Amazon Verified Purchaser of *The One-Minute Cure* book

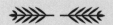

All Health Problems Disappearing

"I've been on the hydrogen peroxide for almost four months now and all of my health problems are disappearing fast. About a month and a half ago my edema came out again in my legs. Today that has all disappeared, I have no more swelling in my legs and the lesions on my right leg that came out at that time will be totally gone in the next few days. I have regained all of the strength that I had completely lost. During the month of December 2010, I made a move to another apartment and I hauled with a trawler boxes upon boxes three flight of stairs throughout the month of December. Before I could hardly put one foot in front of the other. Unbelievable!" -- Email from Claude B., purchaser of *The One-Minute Cure* book

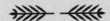

Squamous Skin Cancer Gone in 24 to 48 Hours, Emphysema, Abscess and Plantar Warts Gone, Too!

G'day, I have read your book in the online version, and I could not agree more about Hydrogen Peroxide--"the poison" as most doctors will tell you. I had a **squamous skin cancer** ... diagnosed by a skin specialist. The doctor fixed it by freezing since it was only a superficial cancer. Well, I've had at least 12 more episodes of the cancer since then and I treated them all with 3% food-grade H2O2— and they **dropped off after 24 to 48 hours.** I regularly wipe 3% across my ears and exposed skin to ensure they remain clear. Anything suspicious thing on my skin gets a wipe as well. I drink around 1 mil diluted in 250 mils of water on a daily basis. I have been a smoker for over 50 years-- and **emphysema** tried to get a foothold. The HP stopped the emphysema dead in its tracks. I have had an abscess on one tooth for a couple of years—again, the HP keeps it dormant. Whenever it flares up, the HP stops it again. The 35% works really well on plantar warts, my daughter had one and the HP really cleared it up. I could not recommend it enough from my personal experience as a user of it.

Yours sincerely, Keith Clampett, Australia

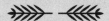

Epileptic Seizures Halted

"We recently purchased your book and I have to say the peroxide therapy is amazing. My son is epileptic and it was totally out of control for the past 25 years. Grand mal activity every 2 weeks. He has been taking the H_2O_2 for a month and not had seizure activity!!! At this time he is also weaning off yet another medication that didn't work—and still no seizure activity.

"My son also has, due to so many seizures, what is called Dupuytens contracture, where his hand bends and he is unable to use. However, with this therapy we have noticed that he frequently has been responsive with this hand and is getting use out of it. I can't wait to see what happens when he gets to 25 drops!!

"Thanks so much for this info. I cannot tell you how

much things have changed!!" - - Michele D., Amazon
Verified Purchaser of *The One-Minute Cure* book

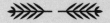

"Super Human!"

"I've been taking H_2O_2 since October 2008 after reading The One-Minute Cure book. I get a complete checkup each year around my birthday, and apparently I have 'super human' low cholesterol. I eat out a lot and fast food and all that unhealthy stuff. But with the triglycerides I'm almost 100 points under the 'normal.' And all my other numbers are 'good' to 'super good.' too." – K. Parker, Colorado

Morning Stiffness, Depression and Dental Abscess — All Things of the Past!

"I'm reporting to you a huge success story of using food grade hydrogen peroxide detoxification regimen recommended in your book, *The One Minute Cure*. I am a 56 year old male. I have had a crowned back upper tooth that has been becoming more and more pressure sensitive to chewing even gum. One month into the regimen I noticed that the pressure sensitivity had dramatically waned and two weeks later it is virtually gone!!!! Well, what that tells me I had an abscess brewing and would soon have been in need of a visit to an expensive dentist chair trip.

Also I have stopped taking anti-depressant medication as I have been feeling in the best mood in years, can think clearly and make decisions and handle stress like never before!

I was starting to have trouble getting out of bed due to stiffness in my knees and pressure sensitive weight on my feet. It would take me 5 to 10 minutes of stretching and slowly limbering up. Not anymore! I roll out of bed with NO STIFFNESS! Wow! I am amazed! -- R. Kennedy, Fargo, North Dakota

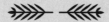

No Longer Need Meds for Heart, Blood Sugar and Cholesterol

"I have read the book—fantastic it is—and already finished the program and am on steady 3x3 a day, feel very refreshed and "living". 1) It cleared my lungs of the "muck" that has been troubling me for over a year. 2) I feel much lighter, I jump up from my chair! I had to use my hands before to help. I bend easily to put on my socks —before my wife helped me with that! I began the program on July 3rd and finished it according to the program. I have been blessed with good health all my life except after my 80th year there were some problems with my heart, blood sugar, cholesterol, etc. according to my doctor, and I have been on meds since. But now I feel as if I can throw them all away! I feel so refreshed! I will be 89 my next birthday in December. Yessir I´m feeling grand!! – Cheers, Jón A. Stefansson, Reykjavik, Iceland

No More Asthma after 30 Years — BPH Problem Gone (No More Meds) -- Forgetfulness Disappears

"My friends convinced me to try the H_2O_2 therapy. I first borrowed *The One Minute Cure* book, and later purchased my own copy. It was so easy to follow the instructions for using H_2O_2 in the book. Easy to understand and put to use. After completing the initial phase, and now on the maintenance dose, here's what H_2O_2 has done for me: **Asthma no longer a problem after 30 years,** no more use of breathalyzers. My benign **prostatic hyperplasia** (BPH) has just about disappeared, and I have stopped using medication for this. As I am 70 years old, I was beginning to feel the effects of old age **forgetfulness**, that has all but disappeared." R. Fornfeist, Montana, Amazon Verified Purchaser of *The One-Minute Cure* book

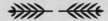

Positive Results with Stamina / Brown Spots / Gray Hair

"I've been on the one-minute cure for 6 weeks now. I noticed that I have much more stamina than before. My brown spots are fading away, and my gray hair has become slow coming in that I now color my hair much less often." – R. Essien, Los Angeles, California, Amazon Verified Purchaser of *The One-Minute Cure* book

~ CHAPTER SIX ~

Hydrogen Peroxide in Nature

Hydrogen peroxide (H_2O_2) is familiar to most people as an over-the-counter chemical compound usually regarded as an oxidizing agent with virucidal, germicidal, antiseptic, disinfecting, deodorizing and bleaching properties. Not everyone is aware that it is also a naturally occurring substance.

A mother's breast milk, for instance, contains high amounts of hydrogen peroxide, and the first milk (colostrum) contains even higher amounts. This has been shown as one of the main reasons why breast milk stimulates an infant's immune system and activates metabolic processes.

Throughout the lifecycle, the human body produces hydrogen peroxide constantly. The immune system uses this naturally occurring hydrogen peroxide to oxidize foreign invaders (phagocytosis)—parasites, viruses, bacteria, yeast and fungus— thereby warding off disease. However, oxygen-deficient bodies are unable to produce enough hydrogen peroxide on their own. That is why oxygen therapy, especially through hydrogen peroxide administration, is extremely important.

> "...The cells in your body that fight infection, called granulocytes, produce hydrogen peroxide as a first line of defense against every single type of invading organism—parasites, viruses, bacteria and yeast. **No other chemical compound comes even close to hydrogen peroxide in its importance to life on this earth...**" —Dr. William Douglass, *Hydrogen Peroxide: Medical Miracle*

The hydrogen peroxide which the body produces on its own helps aerobic (good) bacteria to flourish. It is also critical to thyroid function and the proper development of sexual hormones. All living organisms require certain amounts of hydrogen peroxide to fight disease and remain healthy. In fact, the body's infection-fighting cells produce hydrogen peroxide naturally to kill off every infection possible—from viruses to harmful bacteria to parasites. Its presence is also important for the body's essential chemical reactions, metabolism and immune system.

Swiftly-moving streams contain high levels of hydrogen peroxide; that is why spring water tastes fresher and cleaner. Slow moving, stagnant water is a breeding ground for various types of bacteria because it contains little oxygen. Many of the world's well- known springs, such as those in the Hunza area of the Himalayas and in Lourdes, France, flow with water that reportedly has healing properties. Interestingly, they have been found to have high hydrogen peroxide levels.

Hydrogen peroxide also plays a vital role in nature, and it is especially important to plants. Rainwater contains hydrogen peroxide; this is why plants and grass seem greener and healthier after it rains. In fact, rainwater is much better for plants than tap water, and some farmers have begun adding diluted hydrogen peroxide to the water sprayed on plants. To make them grow bigger and more beautiful, you may want to water your plants with water containing a solution of one ounce of 3% hydrogen peroxide to a quart of water. Seeds soaked in one ounce of hydrogen peroxide mixed with a pint of water grow more quickly and become larger.

Hydrogen peroxide is important for animals too, and it has proven effective in curing feline leukemia. Dogs also benefit from having a drop added to their drinking water, as it has demonstrated the ability to cure distemper. Many farmers have also found it beneficial to add hydrogen peroxide to the drinking water of livestock, in addition to applying it to wounds as an antiseptic. As you begin hydrogen peroxide therapy, you may wish to offer your pets the same benefits by adding a few drops to their drinking water.

Do I Lack Oxygen?

In today's world, many people are oxygen-starved without realizing it. Air filled with pollution and smog, aside from being oxygen-depleted, also inhibits our ability to take in sufficient amounts of oxygen. We breathe slowly and shallowly when taking in polluted air, and as a result, our bodies become accustomed to living with less oxygen. Smog is full of carbon monoxide and other toxins, and the body reacts by breathing more slowly and in a shallow fashion to take in less polluted air.

Our atmosphere should ideally contain about 20

percent oxygen, but in some especially polluted areas, it is as low as 10 percent. As a result, it is virtually impossible for us to inhale the amount of oxygen we need to effectively fight off diseases. Even as we continue to pollute our air, we are also cutting down trees—locally and in the rain forests—at alarming rates. Trees breathe in the carbon dioxide we breathe out, and they provide oxygen in return. Fewer trees mean less oxygen for us to breathe.

Tap water contains little oxygen because it travels through pipes, never being exposed to air. It is also treated with high levels of chlorine, which removes oxygen. In addition, the way we cook and over-process food drastically reduces the oxygen content of our food. Fast food—and food that is manufactured and processed to have a long shelf-life—are oxygen deficient. The over-prescription of antibiotics also has detrimental effects on a body's oxygen level because these drugs, wreak havoc on the oxygen-producing aerobic bacteria in the digestive tract. All of this, combined with the sedentary lives many of us lead, cause a lack of oxygen.

Some researchers even believe that many people who are considered to be of average intelligence are actually functioning at much lower levels because of a lack of oxygen. Without oxygen, a person will die within about nine minutes. It stands to reason that a slight decrease in the amount of oxygen a person receives will have detrimental effects on the brain's function over time. Those people who live in large cities with high pollution often feel depressed, tired and irritable, and these symptoms could certainly be due to continually breathing polluted air and smog. Supplementing a healthy diet and exercise with hydrogen peroxide therapy will provide the brain and nervous system with a boost of oxygen that can help a person think more clearly and be more productive.

One of the most exciting prospects on the horizon is that hydrogen peroxide therapy shows great promise as a way to prevent, treat and cure **Alzheimer's disease (AD) and dementia.** In light of the fact that more than 6 million Americans suffer from Alzheimer's Disease, according the the Alzheimer's Association—and over the next 50 years, the incidence of AD is expected to *quadruple*—the personal, economic and social ramifications of a hydrogen peroxide cure cannot be overestimated.

In addition to dementia, memory loss and Alzheimer's Disease—which are conditions suffered by a significant percentage of the aging population—many senior citizens are plagued by other bothersome realities of getting older as well. Hydrogen peroxide once again comes to their rescue. One patient, who is in his late sixties, found it nearly impossible to get out of bed in the mornings. His muscles and joints were so sore and stiff that he would have to roll out of bed and lie on the floor for a while before he could stand. A friend suggested that he try hydrogen peroxide therapy by spraying the mist through a nasal spray bottle. He began using the spray a few times a day, and after a couple of weeks he found himself able to practically leap out of bed. He was no longer plagued by the aches and pains often considered an inevitable part of aging, and he soon found that he was less frequently visited by viruses and other ailments.

Older people report that hydrogen peroxide therapy

seems to reverse the detrimental effects of aging, and they often feel better than they have in years. Simply supplying the body with a boost of oxygen will provide increased energy and alertness. More and more doctors believe it will prove the best therapy for all age-related diseases.

H₂O₂ is Perfect for Seniors!

"So I purchased this book back in 2013 and started the recommended protocol immediately on Nov 1 of that year. Overall my health, for a 63 year old male was good. However, I wanted to do something to protect myself from disease as I aged into my senior years. I have been doing H_2O_2 therapy since that time with good results. I find it safe to use and have had no problems. H_2O_2 is a very powerful substance and must be used properly. I went through the entire recommended protocol up to 25 drops and back down. As a maintenance level I do 8 to 9 drops once a day. My favorite time to do H_2O_2 is before I go to bed if I haven't eaten for about three hours. Or sometimes I will get up around midnight and take it if I wake up. I have found that I get awesome restful sleep after taking it. If that doesn't work out I will take it in the morning before I eat. You must take H_2O_2 on an empty stomach to benefit from it. So far the benefits I have received from H_2O_2 is I haven't been sick since 2013. A couple of times I felt like something might be coming on and I double up the daily dosage. In a couple of days all symptoms were gone. Then I return to my standard once a day dosage. Just recently had an inner ear infection. Doubled my dosage and added some drops to my ear. Couple of days all symptoms gone! Also I have had some minor arthritis in my finger joints which is now undetectable. I'm now approaching 68 and feel pretty good for an old guy. I still run about 2-1/2 miles 3 to 4 days a week and really believe the H_2O_2 is helping me do that. And again the awesome restful sleep I get when I take it before bed is truly amazing. It's almost 11:30 PM and I just took my H_2O_2 and headed off to bed. Good Night All! I hope this helps you decide whether to use the H_2O_2 therapy. Sure glad I did!" -- Rod Windle, Amazon Verified Purchaser of *The One-Minute Cure* book

Oxygen and Food Consumption

Overeating is a prevalent practice in modern living. The average person eats more food than his/her body can reasonably digest, and the natural aerobic or "good" bacteria in the body are affected. We also tend to eat too much over-processed fast food, which our blood cells must contend with. The main function of blood cells is to distribute oxygen to the body, but our eating habits often cause these cells to act mainly as the body's waste removal system. Instead of supplying the body with oxygen, blood cells must get rid of food waste first. This waste ends up getting stored in various parts of the body.

As we continue to overeat, our bodies never have the opportunity to rid themselves of stored toxins. Also, the foods we often eat are over-processed, thereby containing low amounts of essential fatty acids which are critical to the body's ability to produce oxygen.

This is another reason why, more than ever, oxygen supplementation via hydrogen peroxide is essential.

> "Hydrogen peroxide therapy can help achieve a multitude of therapeutic outcomes that would be unthinkable with a single drug or mainstream medical procedure. When **levels of oxygen increase,** the potential for **disease decreases**." —Nathaniel Altman, *"The Oxygen Prescription"*

~ CHAPTER SEVEN ~

Why the Controversy?

B io-oxidative therapy, which involves the use of medical ozone or hydrogen peroxide, has attracted some controversy because it is not fully understood by the general population and members of the medical community. Some people insist that bio-oxidative therapy should not be used because of the risk of oxidation. Ozone and hydrogen peroxide give up their extra oxygen atom, and this does cause oxidation. Oxidation is what causes metal objects to rust, what causes a fresh-cut apple to turn brown, and what scientists blame for cellular aging in the human body. That's why people take antioxidants—to slow down the chemical process of oxidation.

What most people don't know, however, is that an enzyme coating surrounds every human cell, which makes it resistant to oxidation. Bacteria, viruses and disease microorganisms, on the other hand, have no such enzyme coating and are therefore oxidized on contact with ozone or hydrogen peroxide.

According to Dr. Frank Shallenberger, who is best known in the U.S. for treating AIDS patients with a holistic protocol, both ozone and hydrogen peroxide actually **increase the efficiency of the anti-oxidant enzyme system,** which scavenges excess free radicals in the body. This then further enhances cellular immunity.

Another source of controversy stems from concern over the internal use of hydrogen peroxide. Why? Because it is a chemical compound that is highly reactive and has corrosive properties. While it is true that at the 35% concentration, hydrogen peroxide is a very strong oxidizer—and if not diluted, can be extremely dangerous or even fatal—the opposite is true when it is diluted in the manner previously described for specific therapeutic purposes. Properly diluted food-grade hydrogen peroxide is not only safe to ingest but also produces the numerous healing effects discussed in previous chapters.

Any chemist knows that the concentration of any given chemical compound affects chemical reaction rates and the overall effects of the compound altogether. For example, arsenic is a metallic poison derived from the chemical element of the same name. It is poisonous at full concentration, but as an extremely diluted preparation, it has had a long history of medical use. The diluted arsenic (called *arsenicum*) is routinely prescribed by homeopaths for digestive disorders including food poisoning, indigestion, diarrhea and gastrointestinal problems brought on by eating too much fresh fruit and vegetables, or too much alcohol.

Likewise, 35% food-grade hydrogen peroxide—although approved by the FDA for use in the production and packaging of foods—is toxic for human consumption at that concentration. However, when diluted in a sufficient amount of water, it oxygenates the body in a way that makes the body heal itself and make itself immune to disease. The maintenance dose, of 3 drops of 35% food-grade hydrogen peroxide in 6 to 8 ounces of water, for instance (see Chapter

5), means that the hydrogen peroxide only constitutes 0.104% of a 6-ounce glass of water, or 0.078% of an 8-ounce glass of water. Like most medications, hydrogen peroxide is harmful or even fatal if not used properly or administered in incorrect doses. Unlike most medications, however, it offers a large number of health benefits without damaging the body or producing adverse effects.

Economic Impact

Many avid users of hydrogen peroxide therapy insist that the main reason the medical community refuses to recognize its incredible ability to cure virtually all diseases, is the economic impact it will have. If the general population gains the ability to treat and cure virtually all diseases on their own (through the use of hydrogen peroxide), the jobs of medical doctors and researchers will become unnecessary. Pharmaceutical companies will become dispensable. In short, there is no money to be made by the medical industry or Big Pharma from the widespread use of hydrogen peroxide therapy.

We, as a society, are dependent on doctors and pharmaceutical drugs to control diseases and ailments—and the people who make money from conventional medical treatments want to keep it that way. New treatments are generally laughed at when first discovered because they seem too preposterous to be true. Only after a long gestation period are they embraced by the general population and considered relevant. We are still a long way from hydrogen peroxide therapy being recognized as the cure-all it truly is, and in the meantime, the pharmaceutical and medical industries will continue to get rich while people die from ineffective, unnecessary and dangerous treatment options.

Don't believe the negative hype you are bound to hear about hydrogen peroxide therapy in the coming years. There is an enormous medical and pharmaceutical community that will do anything to ensure that their jobs and enterprises remain necessary, so they will try to convince you that hydrogen peroxide is dangerous and ridiculous—even if it has cured diseases successfully for over 180 years. You will learn the truth from your own experience with hydrogen peroxide therapy, and you will be one of the enlightened few who will help share this treatment method with the world.

Why Aren't We All Using It?

As mentioned in previous chapters, an estimated 15,000 European doctors, naturopaths and homeopaths have been legally using bio-oxidative therapy in their practices—but the number of doctors using these therapies in the United States is estimated at less than 500. This is because information about medical ozone and hydrogen peroxide is deliberately excluded from the curriculum of medical schools. Our current medical education puts heavy emphasis on drug-based therapies instead.

Additionally, medical boards prevent doctors from using ozone and hydrogen peroxide in their medical practice. Some doctors, including the late Dr. Robert Atkins, the physician noted for the Atkins Diet, and author of 17 nutrition-based books, have been threatened with revocation of their medical licenses if they administer ozone or hydrogen peroxide.

Many clinics that offered the therapy have been shut down in the past, and health practitioners have been imprisoned or threatened with jail time for the same reason. Even doctors who simply make a public statement regarding the benefits of hydrogen peroxide (without actually administering it to patients) have been ridiculed into silence, as in the case of the renowned cardiac surgeon, Dr. Christiaan Barnard, who was impressed by the effectiveness, and was himself a daily user of hydrogen peroxide. (See Chapter 4)

Since the 1920s, thousands of scientific articles have been written about the amazing effects of hydrogen peroxide therapy, but it continues to be ignored or called illegitimate. The true reason why hydrogen peroxide is still controversial is due to a political—rather than a health—issue. Consider that the Medizone Company tried to begin human testing to make ozone therapy commonplace in the 1980s only to be halted by the FDA. If the treatment were to be accepted today, the FDA and many others would have to take responsibility for the thousands of people who have died because they caused this vital information to be withheld from the public.

Other countries, like Germany, Russia, Cuba, Austria, Italy and Mexico have already adopted the therapeutic use of hydrogen peroxide with great success. Interestingly, the people from these countries tend to be much healthier—or less encumbered with disease—than most Americans. The bottom line is that economic and political players are going to continue trying to keep us in the dark about the most effective way to cure disease.

As alluded to in the previous chapters of this book,

the controversy surrounding bio-oxidative therapy—more specifically the internal use of hydrogen peroxide—is largely a controversy that is perpetrated by those whose incomes are threatened by the possible widespread use of hydrogen peroxide.

At the time of this writing, pharmaceutical companies have put pressure on the FDA to issue warnings about the use of 35% food-grade hydrogen peroxide for therapeutic purposes. For example, the FDA issued a press release on July 27, 2006 titled, *"FDA Warns Consumers Against Drinking High-Strength Hydrogen Peroxide for Medicinal Use"*. Should you believe it?

Consider this for a moment: The drug companies have representatives on nearly all the committees in the FDA. These representatives are there for <u>one reason only</u>—to protect the interests of pharmaceutical companies.

Therefore, if there is any natural remedy, substance or therapy which may be effective—but has the potential to outsell and outperform a drug company's product, of course they are going to fight to discredit it, or even have it outlawed, if at all possible. This is just par for the course in an industry which will do anything to protect its financial interests. Just imagine what would happen if drugs were officially rendered unnecessary because disease has become non-existent! That would cause the trillion-dollar pharmaceutical industry to come tumbling down. That's why it employs pharmaceutical lobbyists in Washington that outnumber Congressmen 2 to 1.

The Biggest Threat to the Pharmaceutical Cartel

The information in this book represents the biggest threat to the revenues of the pharmaceutical industry—bigger than all the alternative healing therapies, nutritional supplements, natural foods and products combined.

I wrote this book fully aware of the possibility that it will meet with opposition from the pharmaceutical and medical industries. It is not my intention to wipe out the revenues of entire industries any more than it was the intention of the whistle-blower—who exposed the big tobacco companies' profit-driven agenda of ignoring public health by manipulating nicotine with ammonia—to bring down the industry he once worked for. I've written it with no other objective than that of improving the quality of people's lives, saving their lives whenever possible, and freeing them from the tyranny of unnecessary (and expensive) drugs and medical procedures.

Caveat: Be wary of individuals and organizations that operate under the guise of "quack watchdogs" and call themselves so-called third-party independent reviewers of natural health remedies. Although some are well-intentioned, most of them are planted strategically by the pharmaceutical or medical industries to...

- discredit alternative therapies that are gaining popularity (including hydrogen peroxide and medical ozone);

- brand doctors who practice alternative therapies as "quacks;" and

- disseminate fabricated adverse effects from the use of such therapies in order to scare people.

This would be reminiscent of the days in colonial India when the British drug companies hired a news reporter disguised as a doctor to *fabricate* a story about a child who supposedly died of brain damage as a result of taking hydrogen peroxide—all in an effort to get the Indian people to stop using hydrogen peroxide and buy British drugs instead. (See Chapter 4.)

Being knowledgeable about the manipulative tricks and maneuvers perpetrated by the pharmaceutical industry will better equip you to make informed decisions about your health. Don't give in to the scare tactics you will most likely hear. Today, there are no valid reasons not to use hydrogen peroxide therapy. I've no doubt that one day, it will be recognized as the best, most simple way to cure the countless diseases and health conditions that plague humanity.

A World Without Disease

Give a copy of this book to everyone you care about. There isn't a person on earth who cannot benefit from this information. I am optimistic that the information I've presented herein will inspire compassion for those who are sick—a compassion that I hope overshadows the lure of profit. The majority of health professionals are slowly but surely beginning to realize that they themselves (and their own families) have been compromised by pharmaceutical companies and have become victims of a drug-centered health care system.

Until the time comes that hydrogen therapy and ozone become part of mainstream medical practice, you can help others by sharing the information in this book with as many people as possible.

When we work together to disseminate the information in this book, we can finally be freed from having to pay a trillion dollars to the pharmaceutical companies that are doing their best day and night to propagate the illusion and the deception that they are interested in our health when in actuality, they are legally robbing us blind with their drugs—without actually restoring our health. We can finally live in a world where we need no longer be at the mercy of disease, and where we no longer fear the ravages of old age and all the debilitating conditions it brings. Wouldn't that be the kind of world we would want to leave to our children, grandchildren and all the generations to come?

Here's wishing you a life filled with vibrant health and freedom from disease!

–Madison Cavanaugh

~ APPENDIX ~

The Missing Piece in the Healing Puzzle

Much has been said in the preceding chapters about the importance of oxygenating the body, and more importantly, getting oxygen into the bloodstream so that the blood can deliver it to the cells and tissues.

However, there is one critical aspect necessary—not only in healing through hydrogen peroxide or medical ozone, but all other healing modalities, for that matter. This may very well be the *missing piece in* the healing puzzle—and the answer to the question: Why do some people get healed while others don't?

The answer to this question may be one of the most important lessons you will learn from this book. Given the fact that bio-oxidative therapies flood the body with oxygen; and in turn, efficiently deliver that oxygen to the blood; which in turn delivers that oxygen to the cells—and given the fact that a high level of tissue oxygen creates an environment that kills viruses, harmful bacteria, pathogens, toxins and disease microorganisms, while revitalizing normal cells—shouldn't *everyone* be healed?

The answer is yes—but only IF the cells are able **to receive the oxygen** delivered by the blood. When the cells are *open*, they will be able to receive the oxygen, and your body will then be equipped to heal itself. If the cells are *closed*, they will not receive the oxygen and therefore, your body will not be able to heal itself. It's as simple as that.

So what causes cells to close? In one word—*stress*.

I know you think you've heard all you need to hear about stress, but this is an explanation given by a Harvard cellular biologist who has spent his life studying the behavior of cells. And when you get this simple concept, you'll gain a deep understanding of how healing (especially via hydrogen peroxide therapy) really occurs.

In order to sufficiently explain this concept, a brief background of the autonomic nervous system is necessary.

The body's autonomic nervous system (ANS) is comprised of the sympathetic nervous system and the parasympathetic nervous system. Under normal circumstances, each individual cell is under the influence of the parasympathetic nervous system, which governs digestion of food; blood flow to different parts of the body; salivary gland secretion; and the absorption of nutrients. The parasympathetic nervous system enables the organs to function properly. When operating under the parasympathetic nervous system, the cell is *open*—that is, it's able to receive oxygen, absorb nutrients, get rid of waste products—and is breathing, dividing, multiplying, metabolizing and doing everything that healthy cells do. In this scenario, whenever the cell is open, the bio-oxidative therapies work because the cell is **able to receive the oxygen.** The average human being operates under the parasympathetic nervous system *most* of the time.

However, there is the other part—the sympathetic

nervous system, which gets activated on cue. And that cue is stress. When you are under stressful circumstances or in a stressed state of mind, the sympathetic nervous system kicks in and your cells go into the "fight or flight" self-protection mode. The cue that triggers it could be something external (such as a grizzly bear or the sight of your angry boss or spouse) which pushes the panic button in your brain. Or the trigger could also be the emotions you're feeling (such as worry, doubt, fear, anxiety), the thoughts you are thinking, or the memories you're remembering. When your autonomic nervous system goes into the sympathetic mode, your blood flow moves away from your gastro-intestinal tract and skin; your pupils dilate; your heart rate increases; blood gets diverted to the muscles and your whole body goes into high alert. When this happens, **your cells shut down** in preparation for fight or flight.

Most of the time, the body is operating under the parasympathetic nervous system, and only switches to the sympathetic nervous system in times of stress. But if you happen to have a stressful lifestyle, and you operate under the sympathetic "fight-or-flight" mode frequently, your cells are closed and unable to receive sufficient oxygen during those times—whether that oxygen is from the air you breathe, from a hypberbaric oxygen chamber, from ozone therapy, or hydrogen peroxide (taken internally or intravenously). And when your cells are constantly deprived of oxygen, you create an environment in your body that is **susceptible to disease** because disease microorganisms are anaerobic (they occur and thrive in areas with low levels of oxygen). Bear in mind what Nobel Laureate Dr. Otto Warburg once said, "Deprive a cell 35% of its oxygen for 48 hours and it may become *cancerous.*" (See Chapter 3)

According to Bruce Lipton, Ph.D., renowned cellular biologist from Stanford University, author of *The Biology of Belief,* and an authority on bridging science and the spirit, the difference between the closed cell and a cell that is open (i.e., in "growth mode") is that the cell that's in growth mode is **impervious to disease.** When a cell goes into lock down, fight-or-flight mode, that cell is not getting oxygen, not absorbing nutrients, not properly eliminating waste products, and not functioning the way it normally should. If the cell remains in that state for a short period of time, the effects are inconsequential. That's why a small amount of stress in life rarely leads to health problems. But if the cell stays in the closed, fight-or-flight mode for an extended period of time, it becomes a sick cell. The main reason for this is because of the **lack of oxygen.** When you choose to remain in a stressful situation or a stressed-out state of mind, that's equivalent to suffocating your body and depriving it of the element that it needs most to survive.

Is it any wonder why stress is considered *deadly*?

It won't matter how much oxygen you inhale or consume. It won't do your body any good if your cells are closed. This is why stress is deadly, no matter what healing modality you choose.

I personally know a practitioner of Traditional Chinese Medicine who is also a master of the healing art of Qi Gong. When he lived in China, a female American lawyer who had late-stage cancer flew to China to see if he could heal her. He taught her how to do Qi Gong exercises, which have been proven to cure cancer for centuries. After a few months of doing the Qi Gong exercises, she went for a physical examination and no trace of cancer was found. When she told the Qi Gong master that she was returning to the States, he urged her not to go yet because he was aware of the stressful lifestyle she used to lead, and she had not yet learned to distance her emotions from stressful situations. But she insisted, and returned home to Los Angeles and resumed her practice of law. As stress returned, so did the cancer. Even though she continued doing the Qi Gong exercises, her condition deteriorated. She made plans to go back to China, but before she was able to, she died. This story underscores the fact that if stress rules your life, your cells will be sick and remain sick because they're frequently closed and unable to receive or absorb any remedy you provide.

It goes without saying that being in a tranquil or joyful state of mind—free of stress, worry, doubt, fear, anger, resentment, guilt, and anxiety—is the ideal state to be in throughout the day. Some people say it's a challenge to be in that state of mind throughout the day because of their personal circumstances or their environment, but that isn't the case.

Stress is not caused by external circumstances. In his research at Stanford University, Dr. Bruce Lipton was able to prove in the laboratory, that it is *wrong beliefs* which often reside in our **subconscious mind,** that create stress in our autonomic nervous system. These wrong beliefs cause us to interpret our circumstances as stressful, even when they aren't.

Stress is simply an interpretation of an internal image that shifts us over to the sympathetic nervous system, and causes our cells to go into the self-protection "fight or flight" mode. Every person reacts differently to any given stimulus (internal image) depending on the beliefs that reside in his/her subconscious, sometimes referred to as *cellular memory*.

Consider a man named Jim, for instance, who is given a tremendous amount of work at his job. If Jim happens to have destructive beliefs that distort the way he views himself and life, he would find that situation extremely stressful. Those destructive beliefs could be things like the belief that that he is unlovable, or that he is not good enough, or that he has to be perfect in order to be loved. They usually lie in the subconscious mind, and Jim probably doesn't know why they're there. Yet, they cause him to react to external circumstances in a way that creates stress. Another man, Mike, on the other hand, given the same amount of work, may not find the situation stressful at all because unlike Jim, he doesn't have unhealthy beliefs that distort the way he views his circumstances.

Therefore, the key to properly dealing with stress is not necessarily to remove yourself from stressful situations but to neutralize the wrong beliefs that cause you to interpret the situation as stressful in the first place. Although there are beneficial ways to remove stress such as doing deep breathing, yoga, Tai-Chi, meditation, etc.—and they certainly are helpful to practice before, during and after the administration of hydrogen peroxide for maximum oxygen delivery to the cells—**they do not remove the underlying cause of the stress.** Neither do they alter the way you respond to the stress. The next time you face the same situation, you will again experience stress because the wrong belief is still there.

There are therapies available that can identify the wrong beliefs that are the cause of your stress and eliminate them, but they usually come at a great cost in both time and money. But when you consider that stress alone can singlehandedly make you sick (without even taking into consideration diet, heredity, environmental factors, viruses, pathogens and disease microorganisms)—and cause you to stay sick even if you use medical ozone or hydrogen peroxide—it's still worth pursuing the best stress therapy available. No true healing is possible without the effective management of stress.

There is one simple and extremely low cost method of removing the underlying cause of stress without you having to undergo a series of therapy sessions, and without spending any time trying to identify the wrong beliefs that cause you stress. This method neutralizes wrong beliefs and is taught in *The Greatest Manifestation Principle in the World* by Carnelian Sage (www.GreatestManifestationPrinciple. com). The book also shows compelling research about the 2 learnable factors that bring about spontaneous recovery from illness—usually without medical intervention; and reveals a powerful principle which, when applied properly, brings you to a level wherein sickness disappears.

~ Frequently Asked Questions ~

Q. Will hydrogen peroxide therapy cure my *specific disease*?

A. For the list of diseases that have been successfully treated with hydrogen peroxide therapy, see Chapters 4 and 5 of this book. <u>Note:</u> We are prohibited by U.S. federal regulations from claiming that anything other than a drug can "cure" anything. What we can say for certain is that the one-minute cure is a remarkable, science-backed natural therapy that creates an environment within the body where disease cannot thrive. This therapy does not "cure disease per se, but rather, enables the body to cure itself of virtually any disease.

Q. Where can I find sources of 35% food-grade hydrogen peroxide?

A. There are many online suppliers of 35% food grade hydrogen peroxide. Please be advised that we (Think-Outside-the-Book, Inc.) **do not sell 35% food-grade H_2O_2, nor are we affiliated in any way to the online suppliers** listed below:

Wellness Shop Products: www.WellnessShopProducts.com
Email: rockwellfulfillment@gmail.com
Tel: (916) 897-6565

Guardian of Eden: http://www.dfwx.com/h2o2.htm
Email: guardianofeden12@gmail.com
Tel: (352) 563-5200

Pure Health Discounts:
https://www.purehealthdiscounts.com/wholesale.htm
Email: PureHealthDiscount@live.com
Tel: (352) 564-0404

There are many other suppliers of food-grade H_2O_2 that you can find online. Just do a search on Google using "35% food-grade hydrogen peroxide" as your search criteria.

If you live in a city/country outside the U.S., do a search on Google or other search engines under the following search term "35% food grade hydrogen peroxide +YourCity/Country". Don't forget to put the plus sign (+) before the name of your city or country so as to narrow your search to suppliers in your part of the world.

For a list of retail distributors or brick-and-mortar stores that sell food-grade hydrogen peroxide, go to the Retail Stores section of this book (pages 143).

Q. Can hydrogen peroxide therapy be used by pregnant women?

A. This question falls in the realm of medical advice. Since we at Think-Outside-the-Book, Inc. are not doctors, we're prohibited from dispensing medical advice without a license. Therefore, we encourage you to seek the advice of your doctor or a qualified medical practitioner.

Q. Can I take the 35% food grade H_2O_2 together with alkaline ionized, micro-clustered water (such as water generated by Kangen, Jupiter, Gold Fox, KYK and other ionizers)?

A. The hydrogen peroxide therapy described in this book is best taken with distilled water — or if not distilled, then at least chlorine-free water or water that's free of minerals. That's because H_2O_2 is highly reactive to minerals (especially iron), as well as Vitamin C and fats. And that's also why it should be taken on an empty stomach — one hour before a meal or 3 hours after a meal.

Since we at Think-Outside-the-Book, Inc. are not chemists, we're uncertain whether the chemical composition of alkaline ionized, micro-clustered water will react adversely when it comes in contact with 35% food grade H_2O_2.

Therefore, just to be on the safe side, it would be advisable not to take the H_2O_2 and the ionized, micro-clustered water together.

Q. I read *The One-Minute Cure* and I'm confused as to whether I should use the 35% or the 3% hydrogen peroxide. Which concentration should I use and when?

A. The complete protocol for the internal administration of food-grade H_2O_2 calls for a specific number of drops of 35% food grade H_2O_2 diluted in 6-8 ounces of distilled water, and this is detailed on pp. 75-79 of this book. The use of the 3% solution is detailed on pp.83-88.

Q. Can I take the hydrogen peroxide therapy even though I'm also taking an over-the-counter or prescription drug *<OR I'm also undergoing medical treatment, therapy or protocol, OR taking other dietary supplements, nutraceuticals, super foods, green drinks, vitamins, minerals, etc.>*?

A. Whenever you're using another health protocol, supplement or medication, it's best to treat that other protocol, supplement or substance as you would food – i.e., take the diluted 35% food-grade H_2O_2 <u>one hour before</u> it or <u>3 hours after</u> it — so as to avoid any reactions with the reactive H_2O_2. As stated in The One-Minute Cure, the only liquids that can be used to dilute 35% food-grade H_2O_2 besides distilled water are milk, aloe vera or watermelon juice.

Q. If hydrogen peroxide therapy prevents and cures virtually all diseases, would it be okay for me to stop taking vitamins, minerals, herbs and dietary supplements, which I only use as insurance since I don't know whether my diet supplies my body with sufficient nutrition?

A. The hydrogen peroxide therapy described in The One-Minute Cure does not take the place of food or supplements. In order for the body to function properly, it not only needs oxygen but also the proper food and nutrients. If one has a balanced diet that provides sufficient nutrition, then vitamins, minerals and other supplements may be unnecessary. But in this modern world, where devitalized food is the norm, it's often difficult to get the necessary amount of nutrition we need from the food we eat.

Q. Instead of doing the 23-day program described in *The One-Minute Cure* 3 times a day, can I just take it once a day for a longer period of time? [This includes questions having to do with *deviating from the protocol* described in *The One-Minute Cure.*]

A. Based on Madison Cavanaugh's research, the protocol presented in page 79 of this book is one that has yielded the best therapeutic results. Although other protocols of administration do exist and are recommended by other hydrogen peroxide advocates, we're unable to verify whether they would yield the same results.

If you find the taste unpleasant, try diluting the hydrogen peroxide with six to eight ounces of milk, aloe vera, or watermelon juice instead of water. If you are still bothered by a bleachy aftertaste, cut down on the number of drops you put into each glass and increase the number of glasses you drink each day. Or simply go up to the number of drops you can tolerate—and supplement that oral H_2O_2 regimen by also *drinking ozonated water* (see page 52) or *inhaling nebulized hydrogen peroxide* (see page 89), both of which can also super-oxygenate the body and accelerate healing.

Q. Since I don't have a serious disease that I need to cure, can I just go directly to the maintenance dose (3 drops of diluted 35% food grade H_2O_2 administered 3 times a day) instead of doing the 23-day program described on page 76?

A. Since we at Think-Outside-the-Book, Inc. are not doctors, we're prohibited by law from dispensing medical advice or recommending any internal administration of 35% food grade H_2O_2 over and above what's already presented in Madison Cavanaugh's book (with its accompanying disclaimer). It is our **opinion**, however, that going directly to the maintenance dose described on page 77 of this book should suffice for your needs. We encourage you to make your health decisions in partnership with a qualified health care professional.

Q. Is it okay to use filtered or purified water instead of distilled water to dilute the H_2O_2?

A. Purified or filtered water is acceptable to use as long as it's chlorine-free — and free of chemicals and minerals, especially iron.

Q. Is the H_2O_2 protocol described in *The One-Minute Cure* book suitable for children, too?

A. The One-Minute Cure book presents a dosing protocol which is suitable for adults. It doesn't, however, specify a child's dose. Here's what we found about dosage for kids, but please conduct your own research as well. Since we're not doctors, this does not constitute medical advice, and you are encouraged to make your own health care decisions based upon your research and in partnership with a qualified health care professional.

"Finding the right dosage for your younger children will have to use some smart thinking and regulating. Only you know your child best. Always start with smaller amounts when in doubt and gradually build up. My 16-year-old could not stomach more than 20 drops of 35% H_2O_2 3 times a day. For my 11-year-old, I did a maximum of 14 drops 3 times daily and my 6-year-old, 8 drops 3 times daily."

Q. What is the H_2O_2 dosage for pets?

A. For small animals (dogs & cats) add 1 ounce of the **3%** food grade hydrogen peroxide to 1 quart of their drinking water. [Remember: That's the **3% concentration**, not the 35% concentration. Do NOT use the 3% pharmaceutical grade H_2O_2 found in drug stores. For larger pets, adjust the dose accordingly.

Q. I've heard some people and doctors—even the FDA— warn against taking 35% food grade H_2O_2 orally or internally. Some even claim it's dangerous. Is there any truth to these rumors?

A. Practically every single therapy that's taken orally or administered otherwise, has both advocates (enthusiasts) and dissenters (oppositionists) alike.

As Madison Cavanaugh states in Chapter 7, "The drug companies have representatives on nearly all the committees in the FDA. These representatives are there for <u>one reason only—to protect the interests of pharmaceutical companies.</u> Therefore, if there is any natural remedy, substance or therapy which may be effective—but has the potential to outsell and outperform a drug company's product, of course they are going to fight to discredit it, or even have it outlawed, if at all possible. This is just par for the course in an industry which will do anything to protect its financial interests. Just imagine what would happen if drugs were officially rendered unnecessary because disease has become non-existent! That would cause the trillion-dollar pharmaceutical industry to come tumbling down.

Ultimately, you need to weigh everything you've heard about H_2O_2 and make the informed decision that's right for you. We'd be remiss if we didn't provide you with the following disclaimer that our legal counsel wants us to give: You are encouraged to make your own health care decisions based upon your research and in partnership with a qualified health care professional.

~ ~ ~ ~ ~ ~ ~ ~ ~ ~ ~ ~ ~ ~ ~ ~

~ Bibliography ~

As of the publication date of this book, the NIH's National Library of Medicine website lists over 91,000 published studies about hydrogen peroxide. Only a few of the relevant studies are listed below. To see the entire list, go to www.ncbi.nlm.nih.gov/pubmed (enter the term "hydrogen peroxide" in the search criteria)

CANCER

"A Method of Destroying a Malignant Rat Tumor In Vivo", R.A. Holman, Nature, May 18, 1957, number 4568,page 1033

"The Use of Hydrogen Peroxide as a Source of Oxygen in a Regional Intra-Arterial Infusion System", J.T. Mallams, M.D., J.W. Finney, M.A. and G.A. Balla, M.D., Southern Medical Journal, March 1962, volume 55.

"Application of Hydrogen Peroxide Infusion to Maxillary Cancer", Hiroshi Sasaki, Tadao Wakutani, Sikayuki Oda and Yasuo Yamasaki, Yonago Acta Medica, volume 11, number 3, pages 141-149

"Role of Oxygen-Dependent Mechanisms in Antibody- Induced Lysis of Tumor Cells by Activated Macrophages", Carl Nathan and Zanvil Cohn, J. Exp. Med, Volume 152, July 1980, pages 198-208

"Anti-Tumor Effects of Hydrogen Peroxide In Vivo", Carl F. Nathan and Zanvil A. Cohn, J. Exp. Med., Volume 154, November, 1981, pages 1539-1553

CARDIOVASCULAR DISEASE

"Cardiac Resuscitation with Hydrogen Peroxide", Harold C. Urschel, et. al., Supplement II to Circulation, volumes XXXI and XXXII, October 1965.

"Removal of Cholesterol and Other Lipids From Experimental Animal and Human Atheromatous Arteries by Dilute Hydrogen Peroxide", James W. Finney, et. al., Angiology, April, 1966, volume 17, pages 223-228

"Cardiovascular Effects of Hydrogen Peroxide: Current Status", Harold C. Urschel, Jr., M.D., Diseases of the Chest, February, 1967, volume 51, pages 180-192

"Treatment of Arteriosclerotic Obstructive Cerebrovascular Disease with Hydrogen Peroxide", Harold C. Urschel, Jr., M.D., et. al., Vascular Surgery, vol- ume 1, number 2, pages 77-81

GENERAL

"Peroxide of Hydrogen as a Remedial Agent", I.N. Love,. M.D., Journal of the American Medical Association, Volume 10, Number 9, March 3, 1888, pages 262-265

"The Necessary Peroxide of Hydrogen", Robert T. Morris, M.D., The Journal of the American Medical Association, August 9, 1890, page 216

"Some of the Uses of Peroxide of Hydrogen in General Surgery", Thomas P. Manly, M.D., New England Medical Monthly, December, 1892

"Peroxide of Hydrogen", Warren Brown, M.D., The Medical Sentinel of Portland, Oregon, February, 1896

IMMUNE FUNCTION

"Extracellular Cytolysis by Activated Macrophages and Granulocytes - I. Pharmacologic Triggering of Effector Cells and the Release of Hydrogen Peroxide", Carl F. Nathan, Linda H. Brukner, Samuel C. Silverstein and Zanvil A. Cohn, J. Exp. Med., January, 1979, volume 149, pages 84-99

"Extracellular Cytolysis by Activated Macrophages and Granulocytes - I. Hydrogen Peroxide as a Mediator of Cytotoxicity", Carl F. Nathan, Linda H. Brukner, Samuel C. Silverstein and Zanvil A. Cohn, J. Exp. Med., January, 1979, volume 149, pages 100-113

"Hydrogen Peroxide Metabolism in Human Monocytes During Differentiation In Vitro", Akira Nakagawara, Carl F. Nathan and Zanvil A. Cohn, Journal Clin. Invest., November 1981, volume 68, pages 1243-1252

INFECTION

"The Effect of Intra-Arterial Hydrogen Peroxide in Rabbits Infected With Clostridum Perfringens", Bruce E. Bradley, et. al., The Journal of Trauma, Volume 5, Number 6, 1965

"Killing and Lysis of Gram-negative Bacteria Through the Synergistic Effect of Hydrogen Peroxide, Ascorbic Acid and Lysozyme", T.E. Miller, Journal of Bacteriology, June, 1969

"Hydrogen Peroxide Mediated Killing of Bacteria", Dennis P. Clifford and John E. Repine, Molecular and Cellular Biochemistry, 1982, volume 49, pages 143-149

INFLUENZAL PNEUMONIA

"Influenzal Pneumonia: The Intravenous Injection of Hydrogen Peroxide", T.H. Oliver, M.A., B.Ch. Cantab, M.D., and D.V. Murphy, M.B., The Lancet, Feb 21, 1920, pages 432-433

The following monograph was never published in a peer- reviewed journal, but it should definitely be reviewed by anyone interested in learning about hydrogen peroxide.

"The Therapeutic Use of Intravenous Hydrogen Peroxide and its Adjunctive Use in EDTA Chelation Therapy", Charles H. Farr, M.D., PhD., (A Review, Clinical Experience and Experimental Protocol, 1986)

ADDITIONAL REFERENCES:

Otto Warburg, *The Prime Cause and Prevention of Cancer* (with two prefaces on prevention) - Lecture delivered by the two-time Nobel Laureate at Lindau, Lake Constance, Germany, June 30, 1966

Ed McCabe, *Flood Your Body with Oxygen: Therapy for Our Polluted World* - 6th Edition (Miami Shores, Florida: Energy Publications, 2003)

William Campbell Douglass, MD, *Hydrogen Peroxide: Medical Miracle* (Atlanta, Georgia: Second Opinion Publishing, Inc., 1996)

Earth Clinic, LLC, *Hydrogen Peroxide Inhalation Method*, 2008

Dr. David G. Williams, *The Many Benefits of Hydrogen Peroxide*, July 17, 2003

Walter Grotz, *Education Concerns for Hydrogen Peroxide (ECHO)*, Newsletter on Oxygen Therapy, Delano, MN 55328

Peroxide of Hydrogen As A Remedial Agent (Journal of the American Medical Association, March 4, 1988 - Vol. 259, No. 9, page 1279 and March 3, 1988, Volume X, No. 9, page 262-265)

Hydrogen Peroxide Mediated Killing of Bacteria (Molecular & Cellular Biochemistry 49, 143-149, 1982)

Hydrogen Peroxide Release from Human Blood Platelets, Biochimica et Biophysica Acta, 718 (1982) p. 21-25

Killing of Blood-Stage Murine Malaria Parasites by Hydrogen Peroxide. (Infection and Immunity. Jan. 1983, p. 456-459)

Edward H. Goodman, M.D., *The Influence of Hydrogen Peroxide on Hydrochloric Acid Secretion*, Pennsylvania Medical Journal, 1910, Volume XXXIX (Volume XIII, of the Journal p. 339-342)

Interferon (IFN) (Journal of Interferon Research Vol. 3, Number 2, 1983 p. 143-151)

~ Resources ~

Online Vendors - Food-Grade Hydrogen Peroxide:

Wellness Shop Products: www.WellnessShopProducts.com
Email: rockwellfulfillment@gmail.com
Tel: (916) 897-6565

Guardian of Eden: http://www.dfwx.com/h2o2.htm
Email: guardianofeden12@gmail.com
Tel: (352) 563-5200

Pure Health Discounts: https://www.purehealthdiscounts.
com/wholesale.htm
Email: PureHealthDiscount@live.com
Tel: (352) 564-0404

There are many other suppliers of food-grade H_2O_2 that
you can find online. Just do a search on Google using "35%
food-grade hydrogen peroxide" as your search criteria.

Retail stores that sell food-grade hydrogen peroxide:
http://foodgrade-hydrogenperoxide.com/id77.html

Hydrogen Peroxide Therapy Practitioner Directory

The practitioners listed below are Members of the
American College for Advancement in Medicine (ACAM).
According to their online profiles, these practitioners
provide Hydrogen Peroxide Therapy. To find a practitioner
in your area, go to www.ACAM.org and click on the Find
Practitioner tab.

Additional health practitioners (American and international physicians) that practice hydrogen peroxide therapy can be found at the International Oxidative Medicine Association website:
https://tinyurl.com/IOMA-H2O2Practitioners

ALASKA

Ms. Renae Blanton
SVT Health & Wellness
206 Main Street
Seldovia, Alaska 99663
(907) 435-3262

ARIZONA

Laurence Grey
Chandler, Arizona 85225
(602) 999-8118
(905) 725-7000

Kristy Anderson, ND
Mesa, Arizona 85206
(480) 985-0000

Charles Schwengel
Mesa, Arizona 85203
(877) 668-1448

Dr. Ralph Luciani
1530 W. Glendale Ave.
Phoenix, Arizona 85021
(602) 242-4024

CALIFORNIA

Carmelo A. Plateroti, DO,
BPCT
Atascadero, California
93422
(805) 462-2262

Shivinder S. Deol
Anti-Aging & Wellness
Center
4000 Stockdale Hwy, Ste.
D Bakersfield, California
93309
(661) 325-7452
Dr. Juergen G. Winkler
Quantum Functional
Medicine
5814 Van Allen Way, Ste.
212
Carlsbad, California 92008
(760) 585-4616

Howard Press, MD
Carmel Valley, California
93924
(831) 659-2172

Bernard McGinity, MD
Carmichael, California
95608
(916) 485-4556

Frank Shallenberger, MD, HMD
Carson City, California 89703
(775) 884-3990

Hitendra Shah, MD
Diamond Bar, California 91765
(909) 860-2610

David Howe, MD, BPCT
El Cajon, California 92021
(619) 440-7787

Ilona Abraham, MD
Encino, California 91316
(818) 345-8721

Michele R. Raithel
Revolutions Naturopathic
230 Blue Ravine Rd.
Folsom, California 95630
(916) 351-9355

Deepta Saxeena, MD
Fremont, California 94536
(510) 790-2144

Vigilanda Solijon, MD
Grand Terrace, California 92313
(909) 783-2773

Allan E. Sosin
Institute for Progressive Medicine
4 Hughes, Ste. 175
Irvine, California 92618
(949) 600-5100

Joseph Sciabbarrasi
2001 S Barrington Ave. Ste. 208
Los Angeles, California 90025-5385
(310) 268-8466

Jorge L Moreno
Center For Wellness
420 N Montebello Blvd., .300
Montebello, California 90640
(323) 726-6289

Les Breitman, MD
Oceanside, California 92054
(760) 439-9955
Juergen Winkler, MD
Oceanside, California 92054
(760) 439-9955

Dr. Maria Sulindro
890 S Arroyo Pkwy
Pasadena, CA 91105
(626) 403-9000

Andrea Angelucci
San Diego, California 92109
(518) 879-4144

Evangeline Lopez, MD
San Jose, California 95125
(408) 569-8863
(408) 885-0840

Robert Rowan, MD
Santa Rosa, California
95402
(707) 578-7787

Terri Su, MD
Santa Rosa, California
95403
(707) 578-7787

Ron Kennedy, MD
Santa Rosa, California
95403
(707) 576-0100

Salvacion Lee, ND
Studio City, California
91604
(818) 505-1574

Stephen Danielsen, ND
Thousand Oaks, California
91360
(805) 857-0749

COLORADO
Jonathon Singer
Greenwood Village,
Colorado 80111
(303) 488-0034

Alexander Thermos
Lakewood, Colorado 80215
(303)462-1070

FLORIDA
Andreas Grossgold
The Grossgold Clinic
609 Lakeview Rd.
Clearwater, Florida 33756
(727) 330-3844

Chris Enriquez, MD, BPCT
Ft. Lauderdale, Florida
33317
(954) 583-3335

Robert Erickson, MD
Gainesville, Florida 32606
(352) 331-5138

Deborah Viglione, MD
Gulf Breeze, Florida 32561
(850) 623-3836
(850) 934-8138

Tracey Pinkston, MD
Gulf Breeze, Florida 32561
(850) 934-8138

Watson Alternative Health,
MD
Milton, Florida 32570
(850) 623-3836

Jack Young, MD, PhDm,
APCT, H
Mount Dora, Florida 32757
(352) 385-4400

Kirti Kalidas, MD, ND
Orlando, Florida 32819
(407) 355-9246

Kristin L Wulff
Vital Rejuvenation
1462 W Granada Blvd, #220
Ormond Beach, Florida
32174
(386) 238-9872

Ward Dean, MD
6708 Plantation Rd., Ste C1
Pensacola, Florida 32504
(850) 912-6981

John Monhollon, MD
Sarasota, Florida 34221
(727) 399-8600
(941) 955-6220

Alan Sault, MD
Sarasota, Florida 34239
(941) 957-4500
(941) 330-0564

Angela D. Myers
The Medical Healing Center
225 Office Plz
Tallahassee, Florida 32301
(850) 309-1665

Eugene Lee, MD
Tampa, Florida 33606
(813) 251-3089
(813) 251-3096

GEORGIA

Milton Fried, APCT,
ABCMT
Atlanta, Georgia 30360
(770) 451-4857

Winston Cardwell
Atlanta Integrative and
Internal Medicine
45 W Crossville Rd., Ste. 501
Roswell, Georgia 30075
(770) 594-1233

John Virgil Spence
Regenerative Medicine
Associates
1009 East 1st Street
Vidalia, Georgia 30474
(912) 537-0221

HAWAII

Richard Lippman
Honolulu, Hawaii 96816
(808) 373-3034

Alan Thai, MD
Kapaau, Hawaii 96755
(808) 889-5556

IDAHO

Kurt Bailey
Integrative Health
3510 12th Street, 200
Lewisto, Idaho 83501
(208) 799-3333

Stephen Thornburgh, DO
Nampa, ID 83651
(208) 466-3517

ILLINOIS

Terrill Haws, DO
Arlington Heights, Illinois
60005
(847) 577-9451

Robert LaCava, MD
Elgin, Illinois 60123
(847) 695-6262

INDIANA

Randee Miller, MSN, APRN,
BC
Carmel, Indiana 46032
(317) 298 3850

Dr. Clifford W. Fetters
Health and Wellness of
Carmel
11900 N Pennsylvania St.,
Ste. 200 Carmel, Indiana
46032 (317) 663-7123

Linda Spencer, CPNP, FNCP
Indianapolis, Indiana 46254
(317) 298-3850

Dr. Rafael F Cruz, MD
Kentuckiana Integrative
Medicine
405 E Court Ave., Ste. 1
Jeffersonville, Indiana 47130
(812) 913-4416

C. Turner
Innovative Medicine
3554 Promenade Pkwy., Ste.
H
Lafayette, Indiana 47909
(765) 471-1100

Marvin Dziabis, MD, PC
North Manchester, Indiana
46962
(260) 982-1400

MAINE

Alan Weiner, DO
Portland, Maine 04101
(207) 828-8080

MARYLAND

Mark Silvieri, MD
Laurel, Maryland 20708
(301) 490-9911

Paul Beals, MD, BPCT
Laurel, Maryland 20708
(301) 490-9911

L. J. Leo
Today's Integrative Health
6321 Executive Blvd
Rockville, Maryland 20852
(301) 770-6650

MASSACHUSETTS

Barry Elson, MD
Northampton,
Massachusetts 01060
(413) 584-7787

MICHIGAN

David Nebbeling, DO
Lansing, Michigan 48917
(517)323-1833

Rodney Moret, MD, CA
Madison Heights, Michigan
48071
(248) 547-2223

Rick, Ng
West Bloomfield, Michigan
48322
(248) 851-1600

MISSISSIPPI

Rushikesh Mehta, MD
Purvis, Mississippi 39475
(601) 794-3777

MISSOURI

Bonnie Friehling, MD
Columbia, Missouri 65203
(573) 446-1200

David B. Clark
Health+Plus
106 SE 12th St
Oak Grove, Missouri 64075
(816) 690-7377

MONTANA

Dr. Jeff Green
Big Sky Integrative Health
8707 Jackrabbit Ln., Ste. E
Belgrade, Montana 59714
(406) 388-6676

Dan Carter, ND
Bozeman, Montana 59715
(406) 586-2392

John Neustadt, ND
Bozeman, Montana 59718
(406) 582-0034

Christine White
Missoula, Montana 59801
(406) 542-2147

NEBRASKA

Dr. Loretta L. Baca
The Center of Health
302 South Jeffers Street
North Platte, Nebraska
69101
(308) 534-6687

Sarah Kracht
Omaha Health Therapy
Center, LLC
8031 W Center Rd., Ste 321
Omaha, Nebraska 68124
(402) 763-9335

NEVADA

Robert Milne, MD
Las Vegas, Nevada 89106
(702) 385-1393

Thomas Lee, ND
Reno, Nevada 89502
(928) 767-4743
(775) 284-4700

NEW HAMPSHIRE

Julia Greenspan, ND
Hollis, New Hampshire
03049
(603) 249-6783

NEW JERSEY

Scott Greenberg, MD
Cherry Hill, New Jersey
08003
(856) 424-8222
(609) 238-3717

Allan Magaziner
Magaziner Center for
Wellness
1907 Greentree Rd
Cherry Hill, New Jersey
08003
(856) 424-8222

Jeffrey A Weiss
Infusion Center of NJ
842 Clifton Ave., Ste. 4
Clifton, New Jersey 07013
(973) 272-6220

Gary Klingsberg
Center for Nutrition and
Preventative Medicine
177 N Dean St., Ste. 308
Englewood, New Jersey
07631
(201) 503-0007

David Fornfeld, DO
Middletown, New Jersey
07748
(732) 671-3730

David Manganaro
Manhattan Advanced
Medicine
776 Shrewsbury Av, Rm.
103B Tinton Falls, New
Jersey 07724
(732) 383-7310

Stanley Hartanowicz, MD
Toms River, New Jersey
08753
(732) 255-8880
(732) 300-4224

Dante Joa West New York
Healing Center 5300
Bergenline Ave., Ste. 304
West New York, New Jersey
07093 (201) 442-0581

NEW MEXICO

George Keanna, DDS,
FIND, CJN, DANLA
Ralph J. Luciani, DO, MS,
PhD, MD(H)
Lori Eanes, DO
1100 Lead Avenue, SE
Albuquerque, New Mexico
87106
(877) 392-8533
(505) 292-8533

Philomena Marcus, AP, RN,
BC
Albuquerque, New Mexico
87123
(505) 298-1024

Jan C. Jay
Enhanced Wellness
5200 Eubank Blvd NE, Ste
C3
Albuquerque, New Mexico
87111
(505) 323-8100
Wolfgang Haese, MD, DTM,
APCT
Las Cruces, New Mexico
88012
(505) 373-8415

NEW YORK

Gary Jean-Baptiste, MD
Brooklyn, New York 11217
(718) 398-8000

Robert Barnes, DO
Cheektowaga, New York,
14225
(716) 679-3510

Richard Linchitz, MD
Glen Cove, New York 11542
(516) 759-4200

Christopher Calapai, DO
East Meadow, New York
(516) 794-0404

David Borenstein, MD
Hicksville, New York 11801
(516) 749-6447
(718) 758-1650

Michael Schachter, MD
Suffern, New York 10901
(845) 368-4700

Sherry Verostko-Slazak,
ANP-BC
Advanced Integrative Care
8207 Main St., Ste 7
Williamsville, New York
14221
(716) 277-0267

NORTH CAROLINA

Rashid Buttar, DO
Hunterville, North Carolina
28078
(704) 895-9355

OHIO

Theodore Cole, MD
Cincinnati, Ohio 45241
(513) 563-4321

Barbara Singer, DO
Lancaster, Ohio 43130
(740) 653-0017

OKLAHOMA

Gerald Wootan, DO, BOCT,
M. Ed.
Jenks, Oklahoma 74133
(918) 299-9447
(918) 698-7735
Charles D. Taylor, MD
Oklahoma City, Oklahoma
73118
(405) 525-7751

Lance Hightower, DC
Tulsa, Oklahoma 94147
(918) 828-9011

OREGON

Victoria Lutskovsky, ND
Hillsboro, Oregon 97123
(503) 844-6667

John Gambee, MD
Junction City, Oregon 97448
(541) 998-0111
Bridghid McMonagle
Lake Oswego Health
470 6th Street, Suite C
Lake Oswego, Oregon 97034
(503) 505-9806

Jeffrey Tyler, MD
Portland, Oregon 97220
(503) 255-4256

Virginia Osborne, BSN, ND
Portland, Oregon 97223
(503) 805-3438
(503) 697-0725

Terence Young, MD
Salem, Oregon 97304
(503) 371-1558

PENNSYLVANIA

Martin Gallagher, MD, DC, DO
Jeannette, Pennsylvania 15644
(724) 523-5505
Andrew Lipton, DO
Narberth, Pennsylvania
19072 (610) 667-4601

Robert Peterson, DO
Newtown, Pennsylvania 18940
(215) 579-0330
Adrian Hohenwarter, MD
Palmyra, Pennsylvania 17078
(717) 832-5993

TENNESSEE

Stephen Reisman, MD
Nashville, Tennessee 37212
(615) 320-1175

TEXAS

Kazuko Curtin
Austin, Texas 78746
(512) 306-1920

Jeff Baker
Austin, Texas 78746
(512) 306-1920

Jose Saenz
El Paso, Texas 79904
(915) 613-4719

Francisco Soto, MD
El Paso, Texas 7991
(915) 581-2273

Barry Beaty, DO
Fort Worth, Texas 76107
(817) 737-6464

Dr. Gerald R. Harris
7421 Meadowbrook Dr.
Fort Worth, Texas 76112
(817) 457-7177

Joel Mack, NP
Frisco, Texas 75034
(972) 334-9900
(214) 619-1313

John Ferrell, MD
Frisco, Texas 7503
(972) 334-9900
(214) 619-1350

Robert Battle, MD
Houston, Texas 77077
(713) 932-0552

Smart Idemudia, MD
Lewisville, Texas 75067
(972) 420-6777

Patricia Braun, MD
Lindale, Texas 75771
(903) 881-1929

Stephen Dalton, DO
Lubbock, Texas 79424
(806) 792-8843

Melody McClain
Healing From Within
3604 Fairmont, #A2
Pasadena, Texas 77504
(713) 870-5393

Robert Gilbard, MD
Rowlett, Texas 75088
(972) 463-1744

V. John Gonino, DO
Rowlett, Texas 75089
(972) 475-1500

Anthony Rector
Southlake Integrative
Wellness Center
1170 N Carroll Ave., Ste. 100
Southlake, Texas 76092
(817) 329-6263

Frank Setzler
Tyler, Texas 75701
(903) 526-2323
Lynn Jennings, MD
Wichita Falls, Texas 76308
(940) 322-2400

UTAH

Rachel Burnett, ND
Salt Lake City, Utah 84111
(801) 363-8824

VIRGINIA

Leila Zachrison, MD
Fairfax, Virginia 22030
(703) 359-9300

David Schwartz, MD
Louisa, Virginia 23093
(540) 967-2050
Mitchell A. Fleisher, MD,
DHT
Nellysford, Virginia 22958
(434) 361-1896

WASHINGTON

Nazanin Kimiai
Kirkland, Washington 98034
(425) 823-8818

Ralph Golan, MD
Seattle, Washington 98115
(206) 524-8966

William F. Corell, MD
Integrative Medicine
Associates
3424 S Grand Blvd
Spokane, Washington 99203
(509) 838-5800

If you enjoyed this book, you may wish to…
√ Order copies to give away to friends and family members
by going to http://www.1MinuteCure.com
or calling (323) 331-9316. Quantity discounts are available,
as follows:

3 copies = 20% discount
4 to 11 copies = 30% discount
12 to 37 copies = 40%
38 or more copies = 50%
Note: If ordering online at www.1MinuteCure.com,
quantity discounts are automatically calculated after you
enter the quantity you're ordering.
√ Share your comments by sending e-mail to:
Comments@ThinkOutsideTheBook.com